Mayo Clinic
Guide to
Better Vision

3rd EDITION

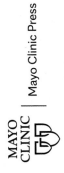

MAYO CLINIC

Mayo Clinic Press

MAYO CLINIC

Medical Editor | Sophie J. Bakri, M.D.

Publisher | Daniel J. Harke

Editor in Chief | Nina E. Wiener

Senior Editor | Karen R. Wallevand

Art Director | Stewart J. Koski

Production Design | Darren L. Wendt

Illustration and Photography | Mayo Clinic Medical Illustration and Animation, Mayo Clinic Media Support Services

Editorial Research Librarians | Abbie Y. Brown, Edward (Eddy) S. Morrow Jr., Erika A. Riggin, Katherine (Katie) J. Warner

Copy Editors | Miranda M. Attlesey, Alison K. Baker, Nancy J. Jacoby, Julie M. Maas

Indexer | Steve Rath

Contributing Editors and Writers | Heather L. LaBruna; Michael A. Mahr, M.D.; Brian G. Mohney, M.D.; Miguel E. Mulet, Jr., M.D.; Cherie B. Nau, O.D.; Gavin W. Roddy, M.D., Ph.D.; Alaina L. Softing Hataye, O.D.

Published by Mayo Clinic Press

© 2021 Mayo Foundation for Medical Education and Research (MFMER)

MAYO, MAYO CLINIC and the Mayo triple-shield logo are marks of Mayo Foundation for Medical Education and Research. All rights reserved. No part of this book may be reproduced, stored in a retrieval system, or transmitted, in any form or by any means, electronic, mechanical, photocopying, recording or otherwise, without the prior written permission of the publisher.

The information in the book is true and complete to the best of our knowledge. This book is intended only as an informative guide for those wishing to learn more about health issues. It is not intended to replace, countermand or conflict with advice given to you by your own physician. The ultimate decision concerning your care should be made between you and your doctor. Information in this book is offered with no guarantees. The author and publisher disclaim all liability in connection with this book.

For bulk sales to employers, member groups and health-related companies, contact Mayo Clinic, 200 First St. SW, Rochester, MN 55905 or email SpecialSalesMayoBooks@mayo.edu.

ISBN 978-1-893005-73-0

Library of Congress Control Number: 2021937317

Printed in the United States of America

Table of Contents

Preface

Think about how much you depend on your eyes for almost everything that you do, whether it's picking out clothes to wear, preparing a meal, driving a car, reading the mail, or using a cellphone, tablet or computer. These daily tasks help maintain your overall well-being and quality of life. So, keeping your eyes healthy and preserving your vision are critical lifetime investments!

Millions of Americans depend on eyewear to correct their vision so that they can see better, resulting in billions of dollars spent each year on eyeglasses and contact lenses. Still, visual impairment can, and does, occur. Dangers to vision include common conditions such as age-related macular degeneration, glaucoma, diabetic retinopathy and cataracts. Accidental eye injuries also can lead to vision loss.

Mayo Clinic Guide to Better Vision, Third Edition is based on the experience and advice of Mayo Clinic specialists in eye health. It provides practical, up-to-date information on some of the most common eye diseases, as well as tips on how to recognize early symptoms and key factors to help you make an informed decision regarding treatment.

The book is written in a clear, conversational style, supported by illustrations, photographs and evidence-based medicine. It's a practical resource for protecting your eyesight — keeping your eyes healthy and your vision sharp at any age.

Sophie J. Bakri, M.D.
Medical Editor

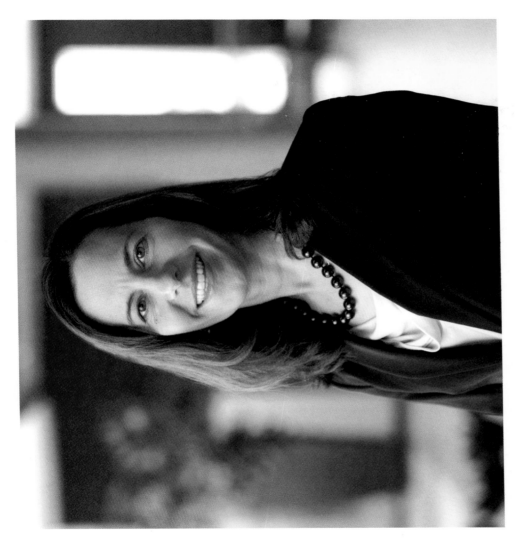

Sophie J. Bakri, M.D., is the chair of the Department of Ophthalmology at Mayo Clinic in Rochester, Minn., and the Whitney and Betty MacMillan Professor of Ophthalmology at Mayo Clinic College of Medicine and Science, an award made in honor of Robert R. Waller, M.D. Dr. Bakri specializes in diseases of the retina and vitreous, in particular, age-related macular degeneration, diabetic retinopathy and complex retinal detachments, including the surgical treatment of these conditions. She has authored more than 180 peer-reviewed papers and book chapters and has served as the principal investigator on numerous clinical trials involving medications to treat retinal disease. Dr. Bakri has received a Senior Achievement Award from the American Academy of Ophthalmology and a Senior Honor Award and Young Investigator Award from the American Society of Retina Specialists.

1

A look inside

For being such a small part of your body, your eyes play an exceptional role in your life. Each eyeball is about an inch in diameter, just a little smaller than the ball used in table tennis. The vision your eyes provide helps you experience the shapes, colors and motions of your surroundings. It stimulates your creativity and apprecia- tion of beauty. It alerts you to danger and the unexpected. You rely on vision to explore, develop, learn and much more.

All five senses are important to you, but sight is the sense you may trust the most when performing many routine activities. With the help of your eyes, you prepare meals, select clothes to wear, read books, write notes, balance bank accounts, drive cars, run errands, perform your job, surf the internet, watch television and enjoy the theater. On an emotional level, vision helps define your self-image and how you interact with others. The author Henry David Thoreau expressed the value of sight succinctly, "We are as much as we see."

Given how much you depend on your sight every day, it's essential to keep your eyes as healthy as you can.

PARTS OF THE EYE

People often compare the parts of the eye to those of a camera, and there are certain similarities. Like a camera, each eyeball allows light to enter its interior through an adjustable opening at the front. An internal lens focuses the light onto a layer of light-sensitive cells at the back of the eyeball, similar to the light-sensitive film used in the camera.

This comparison, however, doesn't do your eyes justice. They have a far more complex, sophisticated function than a camera, or any other piece of technology for that matter. It's not just one but two eyes we're talking about, performing as a perfectly synchronized pair. The materials that make up your eyeballs are extremely flexible, resilient, functional and lightweight.

Each eyeball autoregulates many rapid adjustments for brightness, focus and internal pressure. Light striking the back of the eyeball induces chemical reactions in the photosensitive cells that generate electrical impulses. These impulses trigger two-way communication between your eyes and an optical command center in your brain.

As a result of this communication, your eyes can provide sharp binocular vision and are able to follow rapid movement. All of these features give you vivid, colorful, 3D motion pictures faster than you can blink an eye, literally.

To help you understand vision even better, here are brief descriptions of primary structures of the eye and indications of how all the parts work together. Each structure plays an essential role in the healthy functioning of the eye. At the same time, each structure can be a cause of eye problems.

Sclera and conjunctiva

When you look in the mirror and see the white of your eye, you're looking at the sclera — a tough, white, leathery coating that forms the circular shape of the eyeball and protects its delicate internal structures. The sclera has a single opening that allows light inside the front of the eyeball.

A thin, moist, transparent membrane called the conjunctiva covers the portion of the sclera that's visible and exposed to air. Along its edges, this tissue layer folds forward to also line the inside of your eyelids. The conjunctiva helps protect and lubricate your eye.

Cornea

The cornea is located at the front of your eye, and it covers the opening in the sclera. Comparable in shape and function to the crystal of a small wristwatch, the cornea juts out from the eyeball in the form of a tiny, domed bulge.

The convex surface of the cornea bends the light entering your eye to help you focus on the object you're looking at. The eye's internal lens fine-tunes and sharpens this image.

The cornea, which is made up of several tissue layers, also helps protect your eye. Packed with sensitive nerve endings, the cornea serves as a barrier against dirt, germs and other things that can irritate or damage the eye. When something as tiny as a speck of dust hits the cornea, your brain receives the message instantly. If tears can't wash away the foreign particle, the irritation prods you to locate and remove it.

Pupil

The dark, round spot at the center of your eye is actually a hole in the sclera — like the dark opening of a cave. This hole, called the pupil, is protected by your cornea. It's through the pupil that light passes into your eye, much like the aperture opening of a camera.

Iris

Surrounding your pupil is the iris, the colored part of your eye. Its color comes from a pigment called melanin. The more pigment there is in your iris tissue, the darker its color. Brown eyes have a lot of pigment, and blue or green eyes have less pigment. As you get older, the color may

ANATOMY OF THE EYE

The complex structure of the eye is compact, measuring only about an inch in diameter. Yet in an instant, the eye is able to receive millions of bits of unrelated stimuli from the outside world and relay that information to the brain's visual cortex.

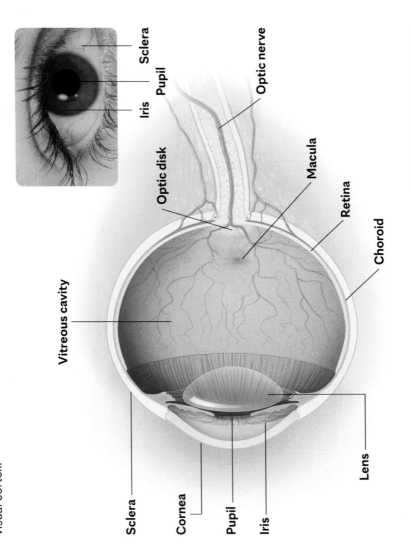

Iris
Pupil
Sclera

Optic disk
Optic nerve
Macula
Retina
Choroid

Vitreous cavity

Sclera
Cornea
Pupil
Iris
Lens

change, as your iris loses some of the pigment.

The iris adds more than color to your eye. It's composed of a ring of muscle fibers that adjusts the size of the pupil, thereby controlling the amount of light that gets inside the eyeball. You might picture this function as similar to adjusting blinds on a window to control sunlight coming through. In bright light, the iris reduces (contracts) the pupil to allow less light to enter. In dim light, the iris opens (dilates) the pupil to allow more light inside the eyeball.

The muscles of your iris react to more than light. Emotions can affect the size of your pupils. Anger makes them smaller, while excitement and pleasure open them wider. Eye specialists use dilating eye drops to get a better look inside your eyeballs during an examination.

The space between the cornea and the iris is called the anterior chamber. It's filled with a clear fluid called aqueous humor that nourishes the cornea and lens, clears waste products, and helps maintain normal pressure in the eye. Aqueous humor is internally produced in the eye,

ADJUSTMENTS OF THE IRIS

The iris adjusts the size of the pupil in response to different levels of light. For example, in bright sunlight, the iris contracts the pupil to prevent too much light from hitting the retina. At dusk or in a dark interior, however, the iris expands (dilates) the pupil to allow as much light as possible to enter the eyeball. In normal light, the average pupil is open a little more than a tenth of an inch.

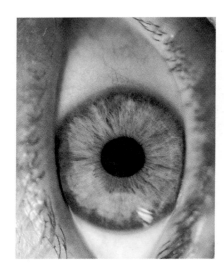

Contracted pupil

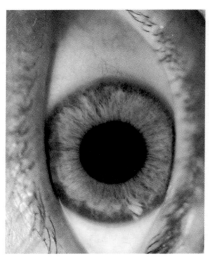

Dilated pupil

and excess amounts drain from the eye through a small opening called Schlemm's canal. The canal is located in the narrow angle where the cornea and iris meet.

Lens

The lens, located directly behind the pupil, is a clear, elliptical structure that helps focus and refract the stream of light entering your eyeball. It's about the size and shape of an M&M's candy.

Surrounding the lens are ciliary muscles. The curvature of the lens changes when the muscles relax or contract. To focus on an object nearby, the muscles contract and the elastic lens becomes thicker in the middle. To focus on an object far away, the muscles relax and the lens becomes thinner and flatter.

These adjustments (accommodations) allow the lens to change its focusing power and sharpen the definition of objects at any distance. The variable focusing power of the lens fine-tunes the fixed focusing power of the cornea. As you get older, your lens loses some elasticity, making it more difficult to focus on objects that are close-up.

Vitreous cavity

The vitreous cavity is the space inside the eyeball that separates the lens from the retina. The cavity is filled with vitreous humor — simply called the vitreous — a substance that's about 99% water mixed with chemicals, giving it a jellylike

consistency. Together with the aqueous humor, the vitreous helps maintain the shape of the eyeball.

The vitreous is clear, so light can pass through it to the retina. You may occasionally notice what look like tiny bits of string or lint floating or darting across your field of vision. These bits are called floaters, and they're condensed strands of vitreous or pigment. A sudden onset of floaters in your line of sight, especially when associated with flashing lights or

ACCOMMODATION OF THE LENS

Changes in the shape of the lens accommodate distance vision (solid line) and close-up vision (dashed line). The thicker the lens, the more that light is refracted and the better the eye can see objects close-up.

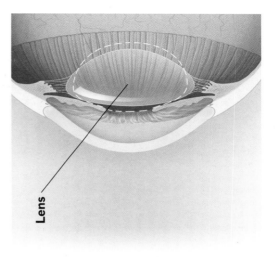

Lens

hazy vision, may mean a potentially serious eye problem.

Retina

A thin layer of tissue called the retina lines the inside wall at the back of your eyeball. The term *retina* comes from a Latin word meaning "net." It's an apt name because your retina consists of millions of photosensitive cells that capture light focused onto them by your cornea and lens, and help turn that light into visual images.

The cells, sometimes called photoreceptors, can be either rods or cones. The two types of cells react to different wavelengths of light.

Rod cells allow you to see in very dim light or off to the side while looking straight ahead — your side, or peripheral, vision — but they can't distinguish colors. Cone cells distinguish color exquisitely but require more light to function. That's why it can be hard to see color in the evening or in dim light.

There are about 20 rod cells for every one cone cell on the retina. Cone cells are concentrated in the center of your retina, allowing you to see the sharpest details when you're looking straight ahead at a well-lit object.

20/20 VISION

It's great when an eye doctor says that you have 20/20 vision. However, that doesn't mean that you have perfect vision. It simply means that you can see objects clearly from 20 feet away — similar to what an average of people with normal sight can see clearly from 20 feet away. The term *20/20 vision* refers to your visual acuity — a measure of how sharply or clearly you can see something from a certain distance.

If you're nearsighted and have 20/50 vision, distant objects will look blurry and indistinct. In fact, they'll look so blurry that what you can see well from 20 feet away is what people with normal vision generally can see well from 50 feet away. Some people have sharper vision than 20/20. Some have 20/15 vision, or even 20/10.

Many factors other than visual acuity affect your ability to see well. Even if you can see what you should from 20 feet away, your doctor will also check for other factors that can affect your vision. These include your depth perception, color vision, contrast sensitivity, peripheral vision and ability to focus on close objects.

Light striking the rods and cones triggers a chemical reaction. This reaction generates electrical impulses that are relayed through the optic nerve to the seeing portion of your brain (visual cortex) and processed there.

The image generated from the light your retina receives is upside-down. It's also reversed, similar to how you see a reversed image of yourself when you look in a mirror. The convex shapes of the cornea and lens cause these effects. Your brain reinterprets this information, allowing you to see an image in its correct orientation.

RETINA

A healthy retina has an even reddish hue. The optic disk is the yellowish-orange circle with blood vessels radiating from it (arrow A). The macula is the deep red spot near the center of the retina (arrow B).

The choroid is a layer of small arteries and veins sandwiched between the retina and the sclera that nourishes the outer portion of the retina. The inner portion of the retina is supplied by an intricate network of retinal blood vessels originating from the optic nerve.

Macula and fovea

The macula resembles a dark reddish patch at the center of your retina. It's densely packed with cone cells and has only a few rod cells. The highly sensitive macula provides your central vision and allows you to see fine detail when you're reading and doing other forms of close-up work.

Located within the macula is a small depression called the fovea. This area contains only cone cells and provides your sharpest vision.

Optic nerve

After visual information is converted into electrical impulses by photoreceptor cells on your retina, the impulses are carried to the brain through the optic nerve. The optic nerve is a dense bundle of more than 1 million nerve fibers, a communication cable connecting your eyes to your brain.

When visual information arrives in the brain, the visual cortex quickly decodes

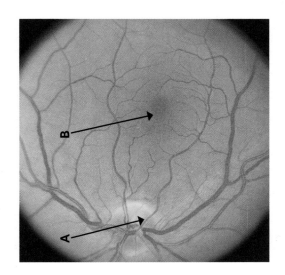

the impulses, coordinating signals from both eyes to produce a clear, 3D image that you can comprehend.

A yellowish-orange circle that's visible on the retina indicates where the optic nerve forms at the back of the eye (see photo on page 15). This location is commonly known as the optic disk.

EYE SOCKET

The eye socket (orbit) is a cone-shaped cavity protecting the eye that's formed by separate structures of heavy bone. The socket is padded with fatty tissue, which allows the eye to move easily. Six muscles control eye movement: up, down, right, left and the twisting motion of the eye when you tilt your head.

Muscles of the eyeball

Six muscles are attached to the sclera of each eyeball. These muscles allow you to

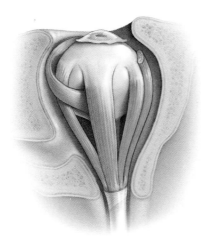

move both eyes up and down and side to side. The eye muscles can work individually or together, allowing you to track an object without necessarily having to turn your head. Your brain coordinates these movements so that both eyes move in unison.

Orbit

Each eyeball is cradled in a socket (orbit) formed by a protective structure of heavy bone. This structure includes the cheekbone, forehead bone, temple bone and bridge of your nose.

Unlike most other bones in your body, these eye protectors typically don't weaken and thin with age. The orbit remains a solid structure. Fat, muscle and other kinds of tissue cushion the eyeball within the orbit.

Upper and lower eyelids help protect the front of the eyeball. By narrowing or closing the opening to the orbit, the eyelids can block debris, irritants and bright light that can damage your eyes. The eyelids also lubricate your eye with each blink. Blinking washes away dirt, pollen and other particles. The lubricant, familiar to you as tears, comes from tear glands located above each eye.

When something irritates your eye, such as chemical vapor from an onion that you're peeling, the tear glands open up. If the tearing is slight, fluid will drain through tiny ducts within each eyelid and into your nose, taking the irritants with it. However, this drainage system can't handle fully opened tear glands. That's when tears overflow the eyelids and they run down your cheeks, such as when you're crying.

CHANGES WITH AGE

Your vision typically changes as you get older. Many adults first notice these changes in their early to mid-40s, when they start having problems reading print at close distance. Many of the changes are more annoyances than obstacles, and you gradually adjust to them.

Here are some ways your eyes change with age, and how the changes can affect your vision:

- **The lenses in your eyes begin to cloud, causing a decrease in visual acuity.** This is known as cataracts. Colors start to become dimmer. Glare forms when light shines directly at you, causing you to avoid night driving.
- **Your lenses become less elastic and flexible.** They lose their ability to focus on objects close by — a common condition called presbyopia. Your night vision also decreases. Less elasticity in the lens may require you to continually change your reading glasses or keep a magnifying glass handy for reading fine print.
- **The vitreous in the interior cavity of your eyeball shrinks and fragments.** Debris from this change may produce bothersome floaters in your field of vision. As you get accustomed to them, you learn to ignore the floaters. But if a sudden increase in their number takes place, contact your eye doctor immedi-

ately. The change could signal an emergency.
- **Tear production slows from the tear glands.** The conjunctiva is no longer able to lubricate your eye and keep its surface clean. The cornea becomes drier, causing an uncomfortable, gritty sensation in the eye. Artificial-tear eye drops may help correct the problem.

AGE-RELATED EYE DISORDERS

As previously described, some vision changes naturally occur with normal aging. But certain changes may signal a serious eye disorder, leading to vision loss if left untreated — these changes should not be considered normal.

Terms such as low vision and blindness are commonly used in relation to vision loss. These terms are closely connected but carry different meanings. Low vision interferes with your functional abilities in daily life, and regular eyeglasses or contact lenses can't help you. You simply don't have enough vision to do what you need to do. Blindness refers to more severe impairment, although you may still have some useful vision (see the sidebar on page 18).

Vision loss stems primarily from diseases such as macular degeneration, glaucoma and cataracts. According to the Centers for Disease Control and Prevention, approximately 1 million people in the United States are considered blind, and more than 3 million have visual impairment (low vision). By the year 2050, these numbers are expected to double.

It may seem as if there's little you can do to avoid one of these eye disorders, but some may be prevented. Even hereditary eye disorders can often be slowed through early detection and treatment. That's why regular eye exams are so important.

Age-related eye disorders include the following diseases and conditions:

Presbyopia

With this common age-related problem, the lens within the eye gradually loses its elasticity and its ability to change shape. As a result, it becomes more difficult to focus on close-up objects without the help of corrective lenses, such as reading glasses.

BLINDNESS AND LOW VISION

In the United States, you're considered legally blind if visual sharpness (acuity) in your best eye is 20/200 or worse with the use of a corrective lens. People with normal vision have 20/20 vision. Blindness doesn't necessarily mean sightless — you may still have a limited amount of vision.

Low vision is not the same as blindness. With low vision, your visual acuity with corrective lenses is 20/70 or worse. With low vision, you may still have some functional sight but you're unable to perform many daily activities in a safe, dependable manner. You may require assistive devices or the help of other people to accomplish your daily activities.

Another common term in use is visual impairment. It's a general term that describes a wide range of visual function, from low vision through total blindness. Visual impairment is sometimes categorized as moderate, severe and profound.

Macular degeneration

Over time, the macula — the part of the retina responsible for central vision — can deteriorate. Age-related macular degeneration is the leading cause of vision loss in Americans age 60 and older. But potential future treatment may reduce the number of people affected by macular degeneration.

Evidence suggests that you can help delay the development of macular degeneration. Taking a combination of antioxidant vitamins has been shown to reduce the risk of an intermediate stage of macular degeneration progressing to a more advanced stage. Medications injected directly into the eye also are effective at preserving central vision in individuals with the wet form of the disease. For more on macular degeneration, see Chapter 2.

Glaucoma

Glaucoma is associated with increased pressure inside the eye. When undetected, the condition can rob you of vision — starting with your peripheral vision and eventually leading to blindness. Similar to other eye diseases, glaucoma is expected to occur in a greater number of Americans in coming decades due to the aging of the U.S. population.

If glaucoma is diagnosed early, damage to the eye often can be prevented or slowed, particularly with the use of eye drops that help reduce and control internal pressure within the eye. Laser treatment and surgery are dependable options for treating more-advanced stages of the disease. For more on glaucoma, see Chapter 5.

Cataracts

A cataract develops from the clouding of your normally clear lens. It's the leading cause of vision loss in the world. With age, almost everyone experiences cataracts to some degree. In the United States, approximately half of all Americans have cataracts by age 75, and more than 1 million cataract surgeries are performed each year.

Surgery to remove the cataract and replace it with an artificial lens is a common procedure with generally

excellent outcomes. For more on cataracts, see Chapter 6.

Eyelid problems

Age-related changes in the tissue or muscle of an eyelid may cause an eyelid problem. Sometimes, the problem progresses to the point where it begins to irritate the eye or impair vision. Surgery may be necessary to correct the problem. For more on eyelid conditions, see pages 131-137.

Dry eyes

Tears are essential for lubricating your eyes. Unfortunately, tear production and the quality of tear fluid decrease with aging, often causing stinging, burning and scratchiness in the eyes. There are simple steps you can take to minimize these symptoms. For more on dry eyes, see pages 138-139.

The eye exam

An eye exam involves a variety of tests to evaluate different elements of vision. These elements include sharpness (acuity), central and side (peripheral) vision, depth perception, color perception, and the ability to see detail. All are fundamental to your visual awareness of the world around you.

A thorough exam can evaluate the quality of your vision — how well you see right now — as well as detect potential vision changes and the presence of eye disease. Information gained from an eye exam also helps guide decisions on how to correct vision problems.

During your exam, your eyes may be evaluated with a bright light. You may be asked to look through an endless array of lenses and to read letters of varying sizes on a wall or directly in front of you. You may be asked to look for flashing lights or merging images. Finally, your pupils may be dilated, making your eyes sensitive to light for hours after the exam.

If a problem is detected, the exam can help determine how serious it is. Catching eye disease at an early stage allows it to be treated before permanent damage occurs.

This section describes some of the more common tests. Your exam will be conducted by an eye specialist — an ophthalmologist, optometrist or optician. If the exam is being conducted in a larger facility, more than one specialist may be involved in the exam. For more information on the different professionals who perform eye exams, see pages 164-165.

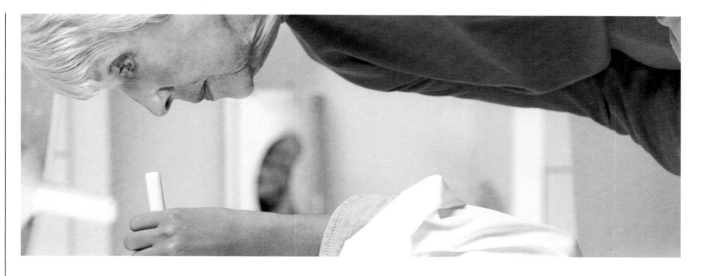

External eye exam

Your exam may begin with an eye specialist asking you a few simple questions. He or she may ask if you've noticed any vision changes, or if you're experiencing symptoms, such as itching, dryness, tearing or discharge around the eyelids. The specialist may inquire how these changes are affecting your vision and quality of life.

Next may come a quick check of your eyes without the use of any special instruments other than a light. The purpose of this is to check:

- Your pupils to see if they respond normally to changes in lighting
- The position and movement of your eyes, eyelids and eyelashes
- The appearance of your cornea and iris for clarity and shininess

An eye specialist may also perform some simple tests to assess the muscles that control eye movement. He or she is looking for signs of muscle weakness or poor control.

In addition, the specialist will study the response of your eyes while asking you to move them in specific directions (up, down, left or right). He or she may move an object, such as a pen, from side to side and ask you to visually track the movement of the object.

Visual field test (perimetry)

Your visual field includes everything you see while gazing steadily in one direction without moving your eyes. Perimetry measures the boundaries of your visual field and indicates whether you may have difficulty with your side (peripheral) vision. There are several types of visual field tests.

Confrontation exam

With one eye covered, you look straight ahead and indicate whenever you see the specialist move a hand in and out of your visual field.

Amsler grid

You focus on a black dot in the center of a grid and describe whether any of the grid lines appear blurred, wavy or distorted.

Tangent screen exam

A short distance away from a screen, you look straight ahead at a target and signal whenever you see an object, such as a wand or a pen, move into your peripheral vision.

Automated perimetry

For this test (shown below) you look straight ahead at a testing screen on which small lights flash on and off at different locations. You respond each time you see a flash.

The automated machinery maps your response to the flashes of light and pinpoints gaps in your peripheral vision. Characteristic patterns of visual field loss on the maps may indicate an eye disorder such as glaucoma.

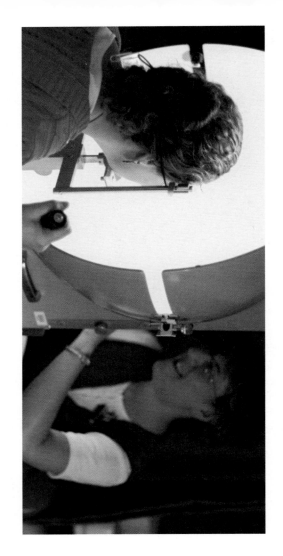

Visual acuity test

Acuity describes the sharpness of your vision or how well your eyes can focus on an object. An eye specialist may test your acuity by checking how well you can read the letters of the alphabet on a standard Snellen chart, positioned about 20 feet away. As you look down the chart, the lines of letters get smaller. Each eye is tested separately while the other one is covered.

You may also be tested as to how well you can focus on objects up close. For this test, you're asked to read the smallest letters that you can see on a card that's held 14 to 16 inches in front of your eyes.

With what's called the cover test, you're asked to look at an object in the room with one eye while the other eye is covered. The specialist observes the movement of the uncovered eye and the amount of time required to focus on the object.

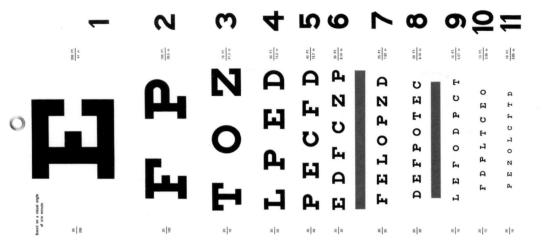

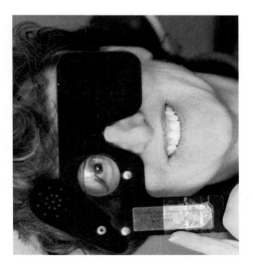

Snellen chart A Snellen chart is a very common component of an eye exam used to evaluate visual acuity. This test is performed to assess how well you can read letters from across the room.

Refraction assessment

Refraction refers to how light waves bend as they pass through the cornea and lens at the front of your eye. The waves bend because they're traveling through a denser medium than air.

The curvatures of the cornea and lens have to be just right for light to focus directly on your retina. If the curvature of either structure is too steep or too flat, the sharpest focus may occur before light reaches your retina (nearsightedness) or at an imaginary point behind your retina (farsightedness).

A refraction assessment helps determine your eyeglass or contact lens prescription to resolve the refractive error. If you don't need corrective lenses, you might not have this assessment.

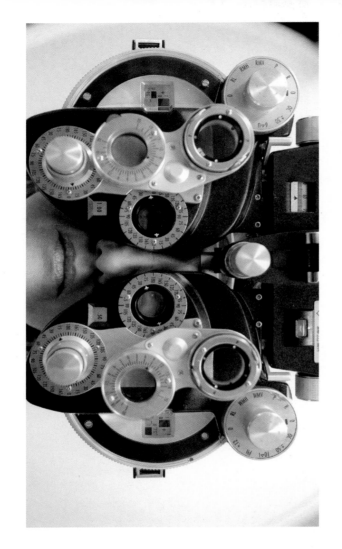

A computerized refractor is often used to measure the prescription you need. Or your eye specialist may make a close estimate of the prescription based on the light reflected by your retina (retinoscopy).

The specialist will likely fine-tune test results with a phoropter. This masklike device contains wheels of different lenses (shown below).

During a phoropter exam, you read aloud the letters on a Snellen chart while looking through the device. As you're reading, the eye specialist makes device adjustments, with the goal of finding the lenses best suited to your vision needs. The specialist will likely ask you which adjustments provide the sharpest vision.

Slit-lamp examination

A slit lamp helps examine structures at the front of your eye under high magnification. The device uses an intense line of light — a slit — to illuminate both a front view and a side (oblique) view of the cornea, iris and lens. The instrument allows an eye specialist to view all of these structures in 3D and detect the presence of small abnormalities.

Before the exam, eye drops are used to dilate your pupils and numb the surface of the eye. In some cases, a camera is attached to the slit lamp for photographs. Special lenses may be added to view structures such as the retina.

Fluorescein dye may be used to help identify corneal problems. The dye spreads across your eye and glows bright yellow when hit with a blue light. The illumination highlights tiny cuts, scrapes, tears, foreign material or infections on your cornea.

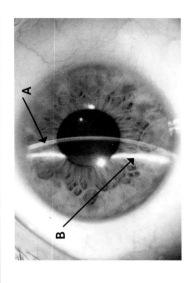

Slit-lamp examination A slit of light is focused to provide an oblique view of the cornea (arrow A). The crescent of unfocused light on the left indicates the surface of the iris (arrow B). An eye specialist can also focus this light for a similar oblique view of the lens.

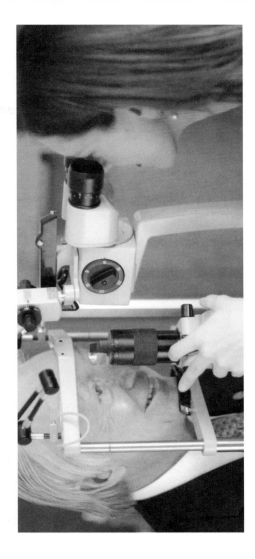

Retinal exam (ophthalmoscopy)

Ophthalmoscopy is a procedure to examine the back of your eye, including the retina, optic disk and choroid. Before the exam, your pupils are dilated with eye drops. Exam techniques include:

Direct exam

Light is shone through your pupil to examine the back of your eye with an ophthalmoscope. This instrument has lenses of different magnifications that allow an eye specialist to focus at different depths.

Indirect exam

For this exam, you lie down or recline. A specialist examines the back of your eye using an ophthalmoscope and a forehead-mounted light — a bit like a miner's lamp (photo at right). This setup allows the specialist to see in greater detail and in 3D. Because of the light's brightness, you're likely to see afterimages, but they disappear quickly.

Slit-lamp exam

While you're seated in front of the slit-lamp apparatus, an eye specialist examines the retina through a microscopic lens and another, smaller lens placed close to the front of the eye. This form of ophthalmoscopy offers the highest magnification.

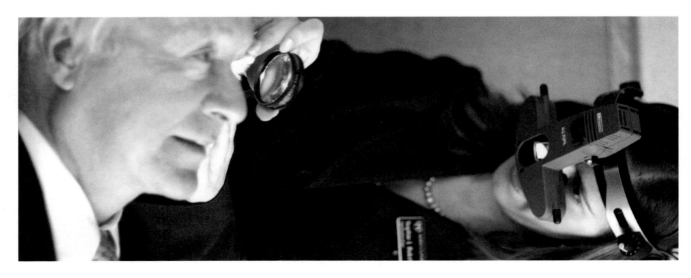

Glaucoma test (tonometry)

Tonometry measures intraocular pressure — the pressure inside your eyeball. This test helps detect the presence of glaucoma, a disease associated with high intraocular pressure that can damage the optic nerve and eventually result in blindness. Glaucoma can be treated if it's caught early. Various methods may be used to measure intraocular pressure.

Applanation tonometry

This test (shown below) measures the amount of force needed to temporarily flatten (applanate) a small portion of your cornea. You receive anesthetic eye drops containing fluorescein, a dye that makes the cornea easier to examine under a blue light. Your head is secured in a support apparatus. While your eye specialist observes, a tiny, flat-tipped cone gently touches your cornea. The procedure

doesn't hurt, and the anesthetic wears off within 20 minutes.

Noncontact tonometry

A machine uses a puff of air instead of the flat-tipped cone to calculate your intraocular pressure. No instruments touch your eye, so you won't need an anesthetic. You'll sense mild pressure on your eye, which may feel a little uncomfortable but lasts only seconds.

Pachymetry

This test measures the thickness of your cornea — an important factor in assessing intraocular pressure. After numbing eye drops are applied, an instrument that emits ultrasound waves is used to measure the corneal thickness.

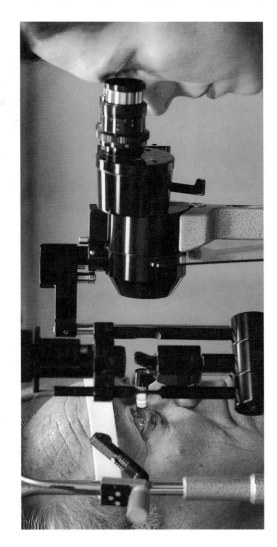

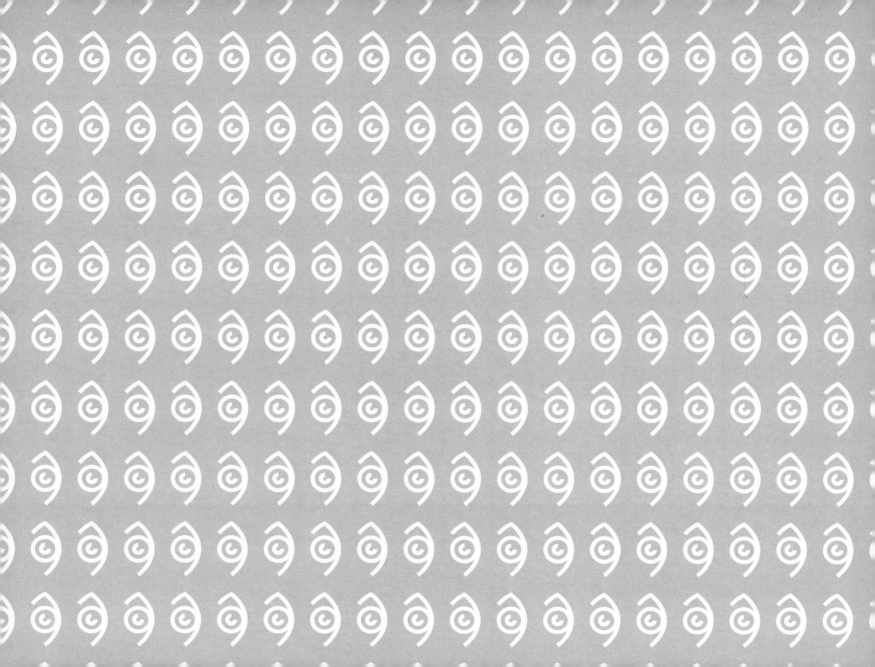

CHAPTER 2

Macular degeneration

Age-related macular degeneration (AMD) is a chronic eye disease that develops when tissue in the macula — the part of the retina responsible for your central vision — begins to deteriorate. The result is blurred vision or a blind spot in your visual field. The disease tends to develop as you get older, hence the "age-related" part of its name.

Macular degeneration is a leading cause of severe vision loss in people age 60 and older. It's estimated that 15 million people in the United States have macular degeneration. As the number of older adults increases, the number of people with macular degeneration is expected to increase as well.

Macular degeneration affects your central vision but not your side (peripher-

al) vision; thus it doesn't cause total blindness. Still, the loss of clear central vision — critical for routine tasks such as reading, driving, preparing food and doing any type of detail work — greatly affects your independence and quality of life. Vision loss may also inhibit your ability to interact with others and join in social functions.

The good news is, a handful of therapies can effectively slow the most serious, vision-threatening stages of the disease, and additional treatments currently in clinical trials are very promising.

THE EYE'S RETINA

The retina is a thin layer of tissue that lines the inside back wall of your eyeball.

It's packed with millions of light-sensitive (photosensitive) cells and nerve cells that capture light focused on them by way of the cornea and the lens, which are located at the front of the eye. The photosensitive cells convert the light into electrical impulses that are sent to the brain via the optic nerve and interpreted as visual images.

These photosensitive cells are either rod cells or cone cells. You need both kinds of cells for good vision. Rod cells are important for peripheral vision and help you see in dim light. Cone cells allow you to see sharp detail and distinguish colors but require good lighting in order to function properly. Light striking either type of cell triggers the chemical reaction that generates an electrical impulse.

The macula is the "high-resolution zone" of your retina. A region that consists primarily of cone cells, the macula is essential for clear visual acuity and for seeing vivid color and detail. A small depression within the macula is called the fovea. The fovea is densely packed with cone cells and provides your sharpest vision.

The layer of blood vessels underlying the retina is known as the choroid. These blood vessels nourish the cells of the retina. The outermost surface of the retina, adjoining the choroid, is a thin layer of tissue called the retinal pigment epithelium (RPE). The RPE helps maintain the structure of the retina and it provides a passageway for nutrients and waste products to move between the choroid and the retina.

SIGNS AND SYMPTOMS

The development of macular degeneration is generally a gradual, painless process, although the disease may sometimes progress rapidly. The changes can lead to severe loss of central vision in one or both eyes if left untreated.

There are two types of macular degeneration: wet and dry. Depending on which type you have, signs and symptoms may vary. They include:

• Difficulty reading printed words, especially small type, because it's blurry
• A decrease in the intensity and brightness of colors
• Difficulty recognizing faces
• Increasing haziness in your overall vision
• Development of dark or blurry spots in your visual field
• An overall decline in visual acuity — how sharply you see detail
• The need to scan your eyes all around to get an intact, complete outline of an object
• Visual distortions (metamorphopsia), such as doorways or street signs that seem wavy or out of whack and objects appearing smaller or farther away than they should be
• Increasing difficulty adjusting your vision to low illumination, such as when entering a dimly lit restaurant from the bright outdoors

With this disease, your vision may falter in one eye while the other remains fine for years. You may not notice any change because your healthy eye does such a

CROSS SECTION OF THE EYEBALL

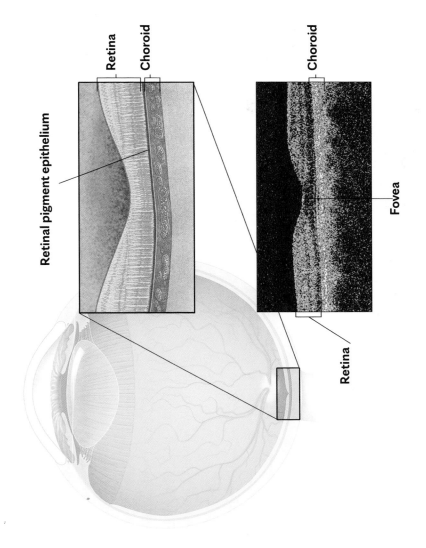

Retina

Choroid

Retinal pigment epithelium

Choroid

Fovea

Retina

The interior surface of the back of the eyeball is lined by the retina, consisting primarily of photosensitive cells that capture light entering through the pupil at the front of the eye. The choroid is an underlying layer of blood vessels that nourish the retina. Sandwiched in between the retina and the choroid is a thin, protective layer of tissue called the retinal pigment epithelium. These three layers are represented in the illustration at top left. Shown at bottom is a form of medical imaging known as optical coherence tomography, which is commonly used in diagnosing eye disease. This image shows a cross section of the retina and its underlying layers, including the choroid. The choroid is the bright red layer beneath the retina. The fovea is the prominent indent on the surface of the retina that's responsible for most of your central vision.

good job of compensating for the affected one. Once the disease develops in both eyes, your vision — and your lifestyle — may be dramatically affected.

Some people with severe vision loss may experience visual hallucinations, such as unusual patterns, geometric figures, animals or even faces. While the hallucinations may be frightening, they're not a sign of mental illness. In fact, these hallucinations are so common that there's a name for this phenomenon — Charles Bonnet syndrome. Should you experience this symptom, you should discuss it with your doctor.

CAUSES

Macular degeneration often occurs following a deterioration of the thin, underlying layer of tissue known as the retinal pigment epithelium (RPE). The RPE naturally weakens with age, and a weakened RPE is associated with the breakdown of vital nutritional and waste-removing processes taking place between the retina and the choroid.

Although the reasons why these systems stop functioning properly are poorly understood, the breakdown may be triggered by a combination of factors.

As healthy, functioning tissue, the light-sensitive rods and cones of the macula continuously shed used-up outer segments as waste. This waste is processed in the RPE and then moved into the choroid for disposal. At the same time, the rods and cones continue to

produce new outer segments to replace the ones they just discarded.

Aging slows the waste-removal system to a point where the discarded outer segments start to build up in the RPE. This accumulation interferes with the normal function of the light-sensitive cells in the macula, causing the cells to degenerate. Damaged cells can no longer send normal signals through the optic nerve to your brain, and your vision becomes blurred.

Blotchy, mottled coloration of retinal tissue and the appearance of waste-deposit clumps (drusen) on the retina are evidence that the waste-removal system is breaking down.

The normal orange-red coloration of the retina will take on an uneven, splotchy appearance as areas of the RPE waste away, often in sharply defined circular shapes (geographic atrophy). The wasting away exposes the underlying choroid layer.

It's not uncommon for small clumps of drusen to appear on the retina as you age, but these deposits generally don't interfere with your vision. Large drusen with indistinct edges are of greater concern. They may merge together, involve the macula and affect your central vision.

A critical development that may trigger more-serious forms of macular degeneration is the growth of abnormal blood vessels within the choroid, a process known as choroidal neovascularization (CNV). Unlike normal blood vessels, the abnormal ones are fragile and easily torn, leaking blood. The accumulating blood and fluid lifts up sections of the RPE.

For a visual analogy, think of tree roots that grow beneath and lift up a slab of concrete within a sidewalk, creating an uneven surface. Swelling and blisters on the RPE caused by leaky blood vessels do much the same, damaging the rods and cones of the overlying macula.

Why CNV occurs isn't understood, but the growth of abnormal blood vessels further complicates other processes that damage the RPE, such as the waste-removal system breakdown. The abnormal vessels may eventually transform into scar tissue, creating permanent blind spots in your visual field.

Scientists have identified certain molecules in your bloodstream called angiogenic factors that cause new blood vessels to develop. One type is a protein called vascular endothelial growth factor (VEGF). There are other molecules in your bloodstream that do the opposite — prevent the growth of blood vessels. They are known as anti-angiogenic factors.

VISION WITH MACULAR DEGENERATION

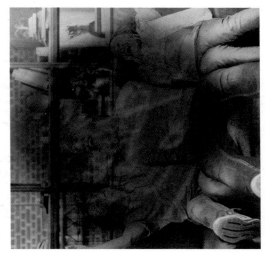

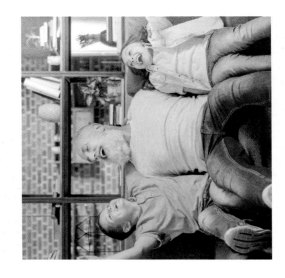

As macular degeneration develops, you may notice a general haziness in your vision during day-to-day activities, including time with family and friends, . A blind spot gradually forms at the center of your visual field. The image at left shows normal vision and the image at right macular degeneration.

Normally, your body maintains a balance between the molecules that promote blood vessel growth and the molecules that inhibit it. Choroidal neovascularization occurs when this balance is disrupted and angiogenic factors exceed and overwhelm the anti-angiogenic factors.

RISK FACTORS

While researchers don't know the exact causes of age-related macular degeneration, they have identified numerous factors that appear to increase your risk of the disease. These factors include:

- **Age.** The prevalence of macular degeneration increases with age, becoming more pronounced after age 65.

- **Family history.** The disease has a hereditary component. If someone in your family has or had macular degeneration, you have a higher risk of having it too. Researchers have identified several genes associated with its development.

- **Race.** Macular degeneration is more common in whites than in other racial groups.

- **Cardiovascular disease.** Studies suggest that a history of high blood pressure, stroke, heart attack and coronary artery disease may put you at higher risk of developing macular degeneration.

- **Tobacco use.** Smoking cigarettes or regularly being exposed to cigarette smoke increases the risk of macular

CHOROIDAL NEOVASCULARIZATION

As abnormal blood vessels grow underneath the retinal pigment epithelium, some blood vessels eventually work their way through the thin layer of tissue and into the macula, where leaked fluid accumulates and destroys the photo-sensitive cells.

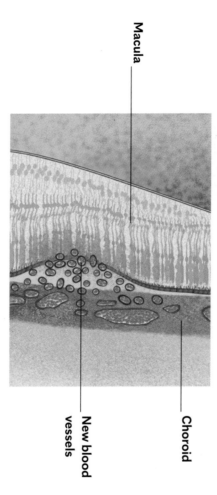

Macula

New blood vessels

Choroid

degeneration. Smoking is the single most preventable cause of the disease.

- **Alcohol use.** Heavy alcohol consumption is associated with an increased risk of early disease.

- **Exposure to sunlight.** It's possible that long-term exposure of your eyes to sunlight may increase your risk of developing macular degeneration, but this risk has not been proved and remains controversial.

- **Diet.** Observational studies suggest that a healthy diet including fruits, vegetables and fish may be associated with a lower risk of macular degeneration.

SCREENING AND DIAGNOSIS

Regular eye exams may detect early signs of macular degeneration before the disease causes severe vision loss. You should consult your eye doctor if you notice any changes in your central vision or your ability to distinguish colors and fine detail, particularly if you're older than age 50.

Macular degeneration, particularly in its advanced stages, may progress rapidly, and the sooner you receive treatment, the better your chances of limiting vision loss.

To determine whether you have macular degeneration, you'll need to undergo a complete eye examination. Screening for macular degeneration includes testing with an Amsler grid (see page 36). If you have an eye condition such as macular degeneration, some of the straight lines will appear faded, broken or distorted as you look at the grid. By contrast, if you don't have an eye disease, the grid lines should appear sharp and unbroken.

Your eye doctor also will take a close look at the back of your eye using either a slit lamp or an ophthalmoscope (see pages 25-26). He or she will be checking for the presence of mottled coloration and drusen on the retina — and in particular, on the macula — as well as the leakage (hemorrhage) of blood and fluid in the macula.

Screening may also include imaging tests, such as fluorescein angiography (see page 50). This exam detects changes in pigmentation or the presence of abnormal blood vessels, which may not be visible with a slit lamp. A similar procedure called indocyanine green angiography may confirm the findings of a fluorescein angiogram or provide additional diagnostic information.

Optical coherence tomography (OCT) is another imaging test that may be useful in making a diagnosis (see page 52). OCT creates a cross-sectional image that clearly shows the layers of the retina and choroid. The OCT image reveals areas where the retina has thickened or thinned, as well as where pockets of fluid have accumulated. A related test called OCT angiography (see page 52) is a newer noninvasive test that examines blood flow and can detect new blood vessel growth.

Although genetic abnormalities are a risk factor for some forms of macular degeneration, genetic screening tests currently aren't used to diagnose the disease. In the

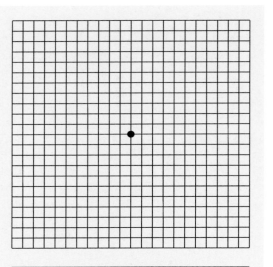

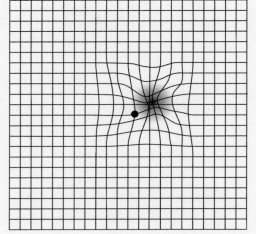

Viewing an Amsler grid in the advanced stages of macular degeneration (right), you may see distorted grid lines or a blank spot near the center of the grid.

Visual symptoms of macular degeneration

You can monitor your vision with regular home checkups using an Amsler grid. This simple test can help you detect changes in your eyesight that you might otherwise not notice. To remind yourself to do the test, hang the grid someplace where you'll see it often — for example, on your refrigerator or alongside the bathroom mirror.

Here's how you perform the test:

- Hold the grid about 14 inches in front of you in good light. Use corrective lenses or reading glasses if you normally wear them.
- Cover one eye.
- Look directly at the center dot on the grid with your uncovered eye.
- Remain focused on the center dot while noting whether all of the grid lines appear straight, complete (unbroken), and of similar darkness and contrast.
- Repeat the above steps using your other eye.
- If any part of the grid appears to be missing or looks wavy, blurred or dark in your visual field, contact your doctor immediately.

future, however, they may be used to assess early risk.

DRY VS. WET

There are two major types of macular degeneration, commonly known as dry and wet.

Dry macular degeneration

Dry macular degeneration occurs when the protective layer of tissue separating the retina and choroid (retinal pigment epithelium) begins to degenerate and thin (atrophy). Dry macular degeneration is characterized by mottled coloration on the retinal surface and the appearance of clumps of waste deposits (drusen). The drusen resemble yellow dots on a color photograph of the retina.

Most people with macular degeneration have the dry form. Age-related macular degeneration almost always starts out as the dry form. Dry macular degeneration may initially affect only one eye, but in most cases, both eyes become involved.

As the drusen and mottled coloration continue to develop on your retina, your vision gradually deteriorates. The thinning of the RPE may progress to a point where this protective layer disappears altogether. This may result in a complete loss of your central vision.

Based on this progression, the dry form of macular degeneration is generally categorized in three stages:

Early stage

The disease is diagnosed as early stage if many small drusen or a few medium-sized drusen are detected on the macula in one or both eyes (see page 38). Generally, there's no vision loss in this stage.

Intermediate stage

At this stage, many medium-sized drusen or one or more large drusen are detected in one or both eyes. You may notice a blurring of your central vision at this stage. Additional lighting may be necessary for you to read or perform detail work.

Advanced stage

In addition to the presence of drusen, the advanced stage involves an extensive breakdown of light-sensitive cells (rods and cones) in the macula, causing a distinct blurry spot to appear in your central vision. This spot may increase in size and become more dense or more opaque as the disease develops.

The size and number of drusen are key indicators of your risk of advanced-stage disease and of developing the wet form of age-related macular degeneration.

Wet macular degeneration

Wet macular degeneration develops when abnormal blood vessels begin to grow underneath the macula — a process known as choroidal neovascularization (CNV). This form accounts for about 10% to 15% of all cases of age-related macular degeneration but is responsible for most of the severe vision loss.

Almost everyone with the wet form of macular degeneration starts out with the dry form. The dry form may turn into the wet form at any time, sometimes rather suddenly and at an early stage. At the same time, it's possible for the dry form to develop to an advanced stage without ever becoming the wet form.

If you develop wet macular degeneration in one eye, your odds of getting it in the other eye increase greatly.

This form of the disease is called wet because of fluid leaking from fragile new blood vessels. The fluid accumulates, forming what looks like blisters under the macula. Eyes with the wet form may also show signs of the dry form, characterized

EARLY-STAGE DRY MACULAR DEGENERATION

The hallmark of early-stage dry macular degeneration is the development of drusen on and around the macula. The drusen appear as yellow spots on color photographs of the retina.

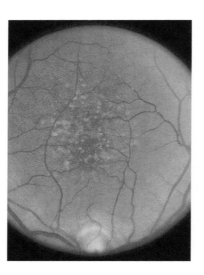

ADVANCED-STAGE DRY MACULAR DEGENERATION

The retinal pigment epithelium at the center of the retina has thinned and disappeared in some areas, exposing choroid blood vessels (arrow A). Large drusen, as indicated by arrow B, surround the macula.

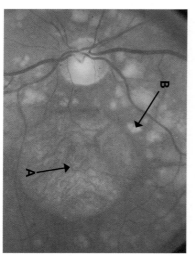

by drusen and mottled coloration on the retina.

Ophthalmologists use fluorescein angiographic imaging to detect patterns of choroidal neovascularization under the retina. The patterns can be used to identify different forms of wet macular degeneration — occult, classic and mixed.

Occult

In this form, abnormal blood vessels and blood from the leaky vessels remain

underneath the retinal pigment epithelium (RPE). The condition progresses slowly and its presence may be disguised by other factors. CNV may have a roughened, speckled (stippled) appearance on a fluorescein angiogram.

Classic

The abnormal blood vessels have started to grow through the RPE, further damaging the macula. The presence of classic CNV is obvious from the brightness of the fluorescein dye on the angiogram.

WET MACULAR DEGENERATION

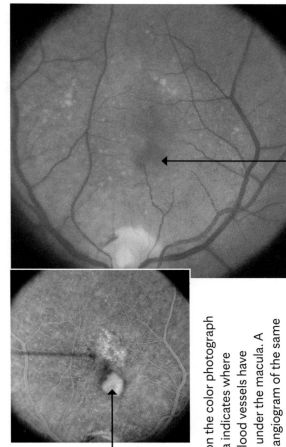

The arrow on the color photograph of the retina indicates where abnormal blood vessels have leaked fluid under the macula. A fluorescein angiogram of the same eye allows the doctor to accurately detect the full extent and the boundaries of the leaked fluid (arrow on black-and-white image).

Mixed

Sometimes, a fluorescein angiogram reveals the presence of both occult and classic patterns of CNV in the retina. This condition may be identified as either the predominantly classic or the minimally classic form.

An OCT scan may show a retinal pigment epithelial detachment (PED), which occurs when blood and fluid leaking from the choroid elevate the RPE, forming a blister or bubble in the macula. This effect may or may not be the result of abnormal blood vessels that have grown out of the choroid.

RETINAL PIGMENT EPITHELIAL DETACHMENT

When the abnormal blood vessels are present, the condition is called fibrovascular PED. Your vision can remain relatively stable with PED for many months — or even years — before it slowly begins to deteriorate.

TREATMENT

In the past, treatment for macular degeneration focused primarily on preserving existing vision and preventing further vision loss. Doctors attempted to slow the disease, but damage to vision that may have already occurred was considered irreversible.

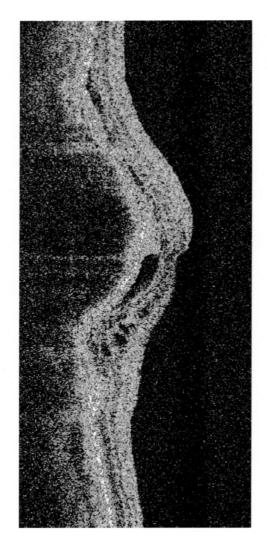

An image of the retina taken with optical coherence tomography shows the elevation of the retinal pigment epithelium by fluid accumulation in the choroid (red layer).

Today, vision loss is no longer considered an inevitable consequence of macular degeneration. New treatments, if administered early in the course of the disease, may repair some of the damage that has occurred and improve vision. That's why it's important to have regular eye exams. The earlier macular degeneration is diagnosed, the better your chance of retaining some functional vision.

In the early to intermediate stages, most people with macular degeneration have the dry form of the disease. Although the dry form has proved to be the most difficult to treat, the risk of severe vision loss with the dry form isn't as high as with the wet form. Because the dry form often progresses slowly, many people with dry macular degeneration are able to continue living relatively normal, productive lives, especially if only one eye is affected.

Although people in advanced stages of dry macular degeneration, or with untreated wet macular degeneration, can experience severe vision loss, that doesn't mean total blindness. While the loss of central vision places severe restrictions on your functional capabilities, you still retain the ability to see light and use your peripheral vision.

If you're diagnosed with macular degeneration, your ophthalmologist may decide on a specific treatment or a combination of treatments to achieve the best results. Make sure you discuss with your ophthalmologist all risks, benefits and possible complications associated with these procedures.

DRY MACULAR DEGENERATION

There was no effective treatment for dry macular degeneration until the release of the Age-Related Eye Disease Study (AREDS), which provided a clear direction for slowing the disease's progression. The study found that a daily supplement containing high doses of vitamin C, vitamin E, beta carotene (often vitamin A), zinc and copper reduced the risk of macular degeneration from advancing to a more severe stage by up to 25%.

A follow-up study — AREDS2 — changed the supplement formula slightly by adding the antioxidants lutein and zeaxanthin and omega-3 fatty acids and removing beta carotene. Scientists then examined the effect of the new formula in halting or slowing progression of macular degeneration.

Study results of AREDS2 indicated that omega-3 fatty acids provided no help in slowing or preventing the disease. However, the addition of lutein and zeaxanthin and the removal of beta carotene from the original supplement formula had positive results. Adding these antioxidants helped reduce the risk of macular degeneration from progressing to more-advanced stages.

For people with intermediate or advanced disease, taking a high-dose formulation of antioxidant vitamins and minerals may help reduce the risk of vision loss. Ophthalmologists recommend using the revised formula (AREDS2) — without beta carotene and with lutein and zeaxanthin added.

WET MACULAR DEGENERATION

A person who starts noticing dark spots or wavy distortions in his or her visual field may be experiencing the onset of wet macular degeneration, the more dangerous form of AMD to your vision. These symptoms are caused by blood and fluid that have leaked from abnormal blood vessels and pooled under the retinal pigment epithelium, elevating small sections of tissue in bubbles or blisters.

Left untreated, the abnormal blood vessels typically grow larger and continue leaking blood and fluid, causing more-severe vision loss.

It's important to undergo regular eye exams to monitor the progression of the disease and to make decisions regarding treatment. Even if treatment can't cure or prevent wet macular degeneration, it can often halt or slow its progression, allow-

ing you to retain a useful portion of your vision. Meanwhile, experimental therapies that may limit vision loss associated with wet macular degeneration continue to be studied.

Anti-angiogenic medications

The growth of new blood vessels within the body is normal. For example, following an injury, blood vessels may form where the damaged tissue is healing. This process, known as angiogenesis, is triggered by certain proteins, such as vascular endothelial growth factor (VEGF), that signal blood vessel cells to grow.

A common approach to treating wet macular degeneration is directed at reducing the formation of abnormal blood vessels. Medications used for this type of therapy are called anti-angiogenic

ANTI-ANGIOGENIC THERAPY

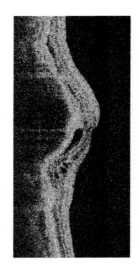

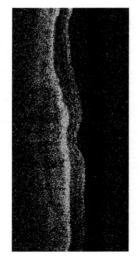

The image at left, taken with optical coherence tomography, shows swelling and the accumulation of fluid in the macula. The image at right shows the same area of the retina after anti-angiogenic treatment.

medications. They work by inhibiting the proteins that trigger vascular growth, such as VEGF.

Anti-angiogenic medications are considered the first line of treatment for wet macular degeneration. The medications are injected directly into the eye and must be administered at regular intervals, often monthly, since the body continually produces VEGF.

Newer treatments in development would allow the medications to work for extended periods — by way of longer acting injections, sustained delivery devices or gene therapies — reducing how often they need to be administered.

Several anti-angiogenic medications may be used to treat wet macular degeneration. They include:

• **Ranibizumab.** Ranibizumab (Lucentis) halts the formation of new, abnormal blood vessels by inhibiting the activity of the VEGF protein. The medication is injected directly into the vitreous of the eye once a month. In clinical trials of ranibizumab, vision stabilized or improved in 95% of participants receiving the medication for a period of 12 months.

• **Bevacizumab.** Bevacizumab (Avastin) is closely related to ranibizumab. It also is administered by injection directly into the vitreous at regular intervals. A clinical trial comparing ranibizumab and bevacizumab (known as CATT) showed that, over a two-year period, both drugs produced similar outcomes when given on the same schedule.

• **Aflibercept.** Aflibercept (Eylea) is typically injected monthly for the first three months, but then may be given every two months in some individuals. Trial results showed the dosing regimen for aflibercept produced similar vision outcomes to those resulting from monthly doses of ranibizumab.

• **Brolucizumab.** Brolucizumab (Beovu), which was recently approved, contains a smaller, more potent molecule than other anti-VEGF medications. A clinical study found it to be similarly effective to aflibercept. The study also showed that after an initial period of treatment, some people may only need injections every three months. However, some side effects have been reported with the medication that are being investigated, including inflammation within the eye that could lead to worsening vision.

A benefit of anti-angiogenic treatment is that it can be used for a broad range of people, not just for those with choroidal neovascularization located outside the fovea, as is the case with other treatments. Anti-angiogenic therapy also is much less likely to cause vision loss.

Medications under study

Several drug therapies are currently being studied for the treatment of macular degeneration. They include medicated eye drops, eye injections, long-acting extended-release drugs and gene therapy.

Clinical trials are in various stages of progress. For an up-to-date list of ongoing clinical trials and for recruitment into new ones, please visit the website *www.clinicaltrials.gov* and type in "macular degeneration." This website is a database of studies conducted around the world, maintained by the National Institutes of Health.

Laser treatments

Laser therapy to treat wet macular degeneration was once a widely used treatment but is uncommon today due to increased use and effectiveness of anti-angiogenic medications.

With laser treatment, a surgeon uses a high-energy laser beam to seal abnormal blood vessels under the macula, stopping the vessels from bleeding in hopes of minimizing further damage to the macula.

The downside of laser treatment is that it causes scarring that can create a blind spot, and blood vessels may regrow, requiring further treatment. In addition, the procedure can only be performed in cases where the targeted blood vessel is away from the center of the retina.

Photodynamic therapy is a form of laser therapy that combines a cold (nonthermal) laser and the photosensitizing drug verteporfin (Visudyne) that's injected into your bloodstream through a vein in your arm. In the bloodstream, the drug concentrates in abnormal blood vessels within the eye. The drug is activated by the laser treatment, causing a photochemical reaction that damages the blood vessels. The procedure may improve vision and reduce the rate of vision loss, but repeat treatments are needed. Photodynamic therapy is uncommon today.

INTRAVITREAL INJECTIONS

Anti-angiogenic drugs are delivered by injecting the medication directly into the vitreous of the eyeball, what's known as an intravitreal injection. This is the most effective way to administer medications to the retina because they reach their target directly. When other means are used to administer a drug, for example, injection through the bloodstream, a much smaller amount of the medication reaches the retina and much larger doses are needed to be effective.

The risk of complications from intravitreal injection is low, and the problems are usually temporary and treatable. The most common side effect is redness and scratchiness of the eyeball. The most serious complication is a severe infection of the interior of the eyeball (endophthalmitis). Other possible side effects include subconjunctival hemorrhage, eye floaters, retinal detachment, intraocular hemorrhage and ocular hypertension.

Surgery

Surgery for macular degeneration is rare. In certain cases when a massive hemorrhage is occurring under the retina, surgery may be performed to remove or displace the blood.

PREVENTION

There's nothing that you can do to change your race or genetic makeup or to keep yourself from getting older — all major risk factors for age-related macular degeneration. But taking the following steps may help prevent the disease or delay its development. The earlier you can begin these measures, the better.

Eat foods containing antioxidants

A nutritionally balanced diet with plenty of fruits and vegetables, particularly leafy greens, may be among the most important factors in promoting a healthy retina. Antioxidant in fruits and vegetables contribute to eye health.

The results of the Age-Related Eye Disease Study (AREDS) indicate that you should include plenty of foods containing antioxidants in your diet. Antioxidants reduce free radicals in the body, preventing oxidative damage to tissues, including those in the retina. Eat foods rich in vitamins A, C and E, including carrots, broccoli, spinach, tomatoes, sweet potatoes, citrus fruit, berries, cantaloupe, mango, whole-grain products, wheat germ and nuts.

Eat foods containing zinc

Foods containing high levels of zinc also may be of particular value in people with macular degeneration or those at risk. These include high-protein foods, such as beef, pork and lamb. Nonmeat sources include milk, cheese, yogurt, whole-grain cereals and whole-wheat bread.

Eat fish

Regular consumption of fish and the omega-3 fatty acids found in fish may reduce your risk of macular degeneration. This has been shown in some studies and in certain populations. Try to make fish a regular part of your diet. Use discretion if you're considering heavy consumption of fish; certain types may contain high levels of toxins and other contaminants.

Take supplemental vitamins and minerals

You may need to take supplements to reach adequate levels of vitamins and minerals in your diet. These supplements can be purchased individually or in combination. But talk to your doctor before using any supplements, particularly in large doses. Unless your doctor instructs you otherwise, don't exceed the Recommended Dietary Allowance (RDA) for any substance.

High doses of supplements may interact with other medications that you're taking, or they may not be right for you. For example, if you currently smoke or you're a former smoker, high doses of beta

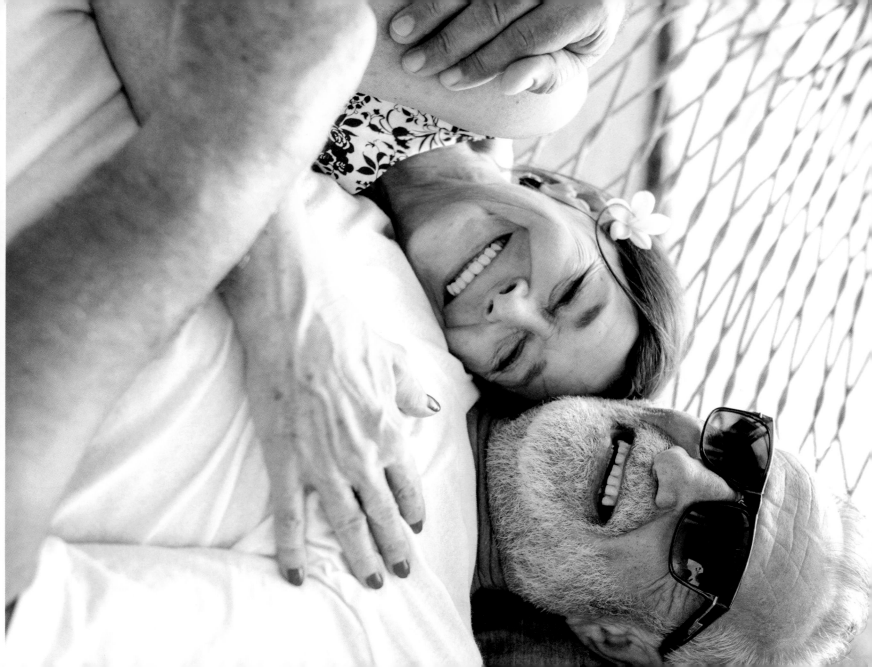

carotene may significantly increase your risk of lung cancer. If you take a daily multivitamin in addition to a specific supplement, check the labels to make sure you're not exceeding RDAs.

Wear sunglasses that block harmful ultraviolet light

Most ultraviolet light is filtered by the cornea and lens at the front of your eye. Still, it's safer to wear orange-, yellow- or amber-tinted sunglasses when you're outdoors. Look for glasses that filter 99% to 100% of ultraviolet A and ultraviolet B rays (see also pages 169-170).

Stop smoking

Smokers are more likely to develop macular degeneration than are nonsmokers. Don't be afraid to ask your doctor for help to stop smoking.

Manage other diseases

The better your general health, the better your retinal health. For example, if you have cardiovascular disease or high blood pressure, take your medication and follow your doctor's instructions for controlling the disease.

Get regular eye exams

Early detection of macular degeneration increases your chances of preventing vision loss. If you're older than age 40, get an exam every 2 to 4 years, and if you're older than age 65, schedule an exam every 1 to 2 years. If you have a family history of macular degeneration, you may want to have your eyes examined more frequently, perhaps annually.

Screen your vision regularly

If you've received a diagnosis of early-stage macular degeneration, your doctor may suggest regularly monitoring your vision at home. You can do this by using an Amsler grid (see page 36). Screening may help you detect subtle changes in your vision at the earliest possible time so that you can seek help promptly.

If you experience vision loss due to macular degeneration, your doctor can prescribe optical devices called low-vision aids that will help you see details better. Or your doctor may refer you to a low-vision specialist. In addition, a wide variety of support services and rehabilitation programs are available that may help you adjust your lifestyle. See Chapter 11 for more information on living with low vision.

Imaging the eye

In addition to the tests included in a standard eye exam (see pages 20-27), an eye specialist may use other tests to evaluate your vision and detect disease. Medical imaging is an essential tool for identifying abnormal structures in the eye and subtle disruptions of eye function.

Imaging of the eye often involves the use of electromagnetic waves or sound waves. The waves are transmitted to specific regions of the eye and collected by special sensors, which convert the information they gather into real-time images. For some tests, special filters or dyes also may be used that help highlight specific eye anatomy.

Sophisticated imaging technologies provide precise visual detail of the structures inside your eye — particularly of the retina and the optic nerve — which can otherwise be difficult to examine.

The types of imaging most often used include color fundus photography, fluorescein angiography, ultrasonography, and optical coherence tomography.

Medical imaging has become an essential tool for detecting and diagnosing a variety of eye diseases, assessing damage caused by the diseases, guiding decisions on how best to treat the diseases, and tracking the effectiveness of treatment.

Color fundus photography

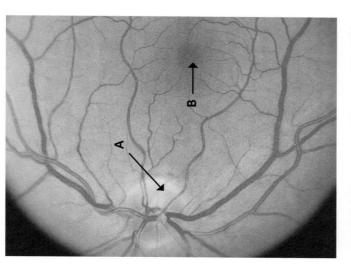

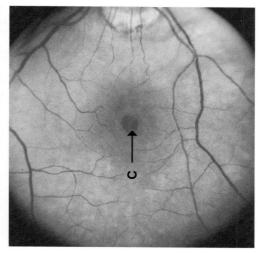

Color fundus photography generally produces very sharp, clear pictures of the retina. The term *fundus* refers to the bottom or base inside a hollow organ. The fundus of the eyeball includes the retina and underlying layers of tissue, such as the choroid, at the back of the eye, which can be difficult to examine.

Color fundus photographs are routinely taken to diagnose a wide variety of eye disorders and to provide a valuable record of change in the color and appearance of the retina.

For this test, you sit with your head resting in the chin and forehead supports at the front of the device, which is a combination microscope and camera. The photographs are taken directly through the pupil opening. Specialized dyes and colored filters may be used for better contrast.

A healthy retina has an even, reddish hue. The optic disk is the yellowish-orange circular structure with blood vessels radiating from it (arrow A). The macula is the darker red spot at the center of the retina (arrow B). The lower image shows the development of a macular hole at the retina's center (arrow C).

Fluorescein angiography

Fluorescein angiography is commonly used to study circulation in the blood vessels of the retina. The test uses fluorescein dye and a special camera that filters out all visible wavelengths except for the dye.

The high-contrast, black-and-white pictures allow an eye specialist to see tissue swelling (edema) and subtle or hidden features on blood vessel walls, such as tiny bulges (microaneurysms) and the leakage of blood and fluid from small tears. The test also reveals new blood vessel growth (neovascularization).

The procedure begins as fluorescein dye is injected into a vein of the arm. After the dye travels through the circulatory system and reaches the blood vessels of the retina, a camera takes a series of pictures, in rapid sequence, which reveals how the dye circulates through the retinal capillaries.

A different dye that's visible under a different wavelength of light may be used in cases where fluorescein dye proves inadequate. For example, indocyanine green angiography provides more detail of the choroid layer underneath the retina.

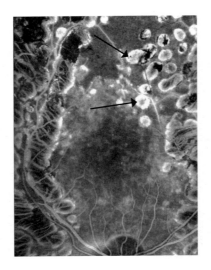

The arrows on this image point to distinct circular formations, indicating the locations of laser burns after treatment with photocoagulation.

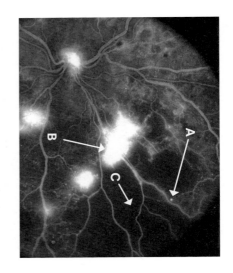

Tiny microaneurysms (white dots such as at arrow A) and leaky, unwanted new blood vessels (clouded spots with indistinct edges such as at arrow B) show the development of diabetic retinopathy. Note also the dark area (arrow C) where retinal capillaries have "dropped out" and blood flow is poor.

Ultrasonography

Ultrasonography (echography) uses reflected sound waves to create an image of the eye's interior in the same way that sonar technology creates images of underwater objects. What's known as an ultrasound A-scan is useful for measuring the size and shape of the eye. The B-scan provides a 2D cross section of the eye and is useful for diagnosing retinal detachments, tumors and eye inflammation.

After anesthetizing drops are applied, a wand (transducer) that emits high-frequency sound waves is placed at the front of the eye (see image below). These waves bounce off internal structures and back to the transducer, which converts the reflected waves into an image on an outside monitor. The wavelengths vary according to the different densities of the tissue that the sound waves strike.

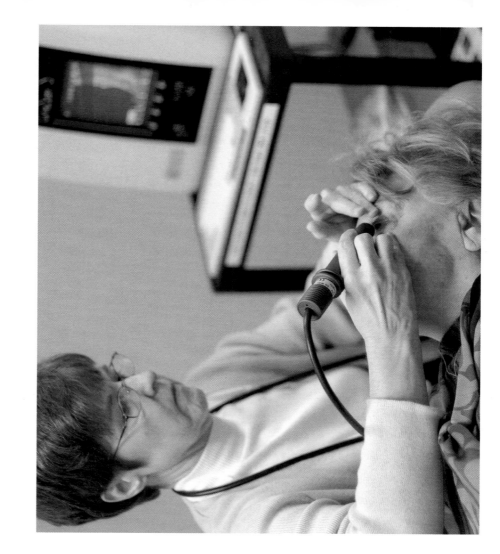

Optical coherence tomography

Optical coherence tomography (OCT) combines the principles of ultrasonography with the high-resolution performance of a microscope. OCT captures infrared lightwaves reflected off the internal structures of the eye, but with a resolution that's many times greater than what can be achieved using sound waves. The result is a detailed cross-sectional image clearly displaying the well-defined boundaries of the retina and its underlying layers.

False colors may be added to assist interpretation, with bright colors such as white, yellow and red corresponding to areas of high reflectivity (greater density) and dark colors such as blue and black corresponding to areas of low reflectivity. The procedure is useful for checking the thickness of the retina and for diagnosing disorders such as macular holes, macular edema, macular degeneration and retinal inflammation.

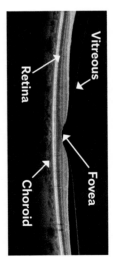

The OCT image above is a cross section of a normal retina. The choroid appears as a layer underneath the retina. The OCT image below shows the results of abnormal blood vessel growth in the choroid. Note the tissue swelling, a pocket of accumulated fluid directly beneath the retina (arrow A) and the dome-shaped detachment of the retinal pigment epithelium (arrow B).

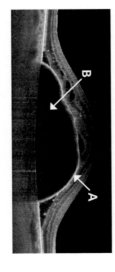

Optical coherence tomography angiography

This is a newer noninvasive method of imaging the tiny blood vessels of the retina and choroid. The procedure is quick and doesn't require an injection of dye into the bloodstream. OCT angiography allows for detection of blood flow and 3D reconstruction of blood vessels. The test is currently used in addition to other tests as it has some limitations. The test isn't yet widely adopted.

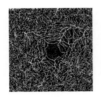

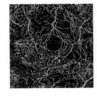

The image at left shows slightly reduced blood flow (black spot) in the choroid. The image at right indicates multiple areas of reduced blood flow (multiple black spots).

Diagnosing disease

When disease is suspected, an eye specialist may employ several types of imaging of the eye in order to get a comprehensive view of the retina and to confirm the results of individual tests.

A color fundus photograph, shown at top, may be the initial image taken during an exam. A dark purplish patch appears on the retinal surface (arrow A), indicating where blood and fluid may be leaking from abnormal blood vessels growing underneath the macula. Small deposits of cellular debris (drusen), which look like yellow spots, are also present on the retinal surface (arrow B).

A fluorescein angiogram of the same retina, as seen in the middle image, clearly shows the boundary of leaked blood and fluid that has collected under the retina (arrow C).

Optical coherence tomography (OCT) provides a different, cross-sectional view of the problem. The OCT image shown at the bottom reveals a pocket of collected blood and fluid that has caused retinal tissue to swell (arrow D), disrupting vision. Also evident is a smaller pocket of subretinal fluid (arrow E).

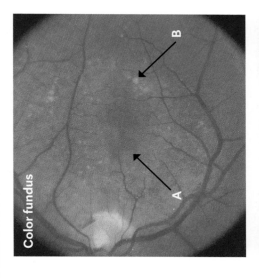

Color fundus

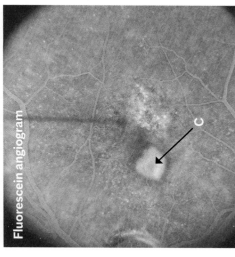

Fluorescein angiogram

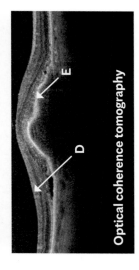

Optical coherence tomography

3

Diabetic retinopathy

Vision loss is a major concern for people with diabetes. According to the National Eye Institute, more than 40% of Americans with diabetes have some stage of diabetic retinopathy. Diabetes also puts you at increased risk of other eye diseases such as cataracts and glaucoma.

The threat of blindness from diabetes may seem scary, but there's more cause for hope than for alarm. With early detection and treatment, the risk of vision loss from diabetic retinopathy — the most serious eye disease associated with diabetes — is small.

If you have diabetes, you can take steps to protect your sight. These steps include getting an annual eye examination and keeping your blood sugar (glucose) and blood pressure under control.

DIABETES AND YOUR EYES

The term *diabetes* refers to a group of diseases that affect the way your cells use blood glucose, which is transported throughout your body via your circulatory system. Glucose is vital to your health because it's the main source of energy for your body. If you have diabetes, you may end up having too much glucose in your bloodstream, and the buildup of glucose can lead to serious health problems.

There are two types of diabetes. With type 1 diabetes, your body produces little or no insulin, the hormone that enables your body's cells to absorb and process glucose. With type 2 diabetes — the most common form of the disease — your body produces insulin, but your cells are resistant to it. When that happens, most of the glucose in your system stays outside the cells and accumulates in your bloodstream.

Diabetes is a systemic disorder, meaning that it affects your entire body from head to toe, not just one area or one organ. Long-term complications develop gradually and may lead to other disabling or life-threatening conditions, including vision loss.

Retinopathy refers to a number of conditions that affect the retina of the eye and may lead to blindness. The root cause of retinopathy may be a disease such as diabetes or high blood pressure (hypertension).

In the case of diabetes, a buildup of glucose in the bloodstream damages the blood vessels that deliver oxygen and nutrients to organs and tissues in your body, including the eyes. The tiny blood vessels (capillaries) located at the back of the eye are often among the first vessels to be damaged.

Capillaries in the retina and macula may swell and leak fluid into the retina, causing your vision to blur. This is known as macular edema. It's a common cause of vision loss from diabetic retinopathy.

Another cause of vision loss is the growth of abnormal blood vessels in the retina. These vessels may rupture and bleed into the eye's clear vitreous, clouding your vision. This is called proliferative diabetic retinopathy (PDR), referring to the proliferation of new blood vessels. At later stages, abnormal blood vessels can

contract and pull on the retina, leading to traction retinal detachment.

The longer you have diabetes — type 1 or type 2 — the more likely it is that you'll develop diabetic retinopathy.

TYPES

There are two types of diabetic retinopathy. Both types can be detected with a thorough eye exam in which your pupils are dilated, making it easier to closely study each eye's interior. Usually both eyes are similarly affected by retinopathy, although the disease may be more advanced in one eye than in the other.

Nonproliferative type

Nonproliferative diabetic retinopathy (NPDR) is the most common form of the disease, as well as the earliest form. It's also sometimes called background diabetic retinopathy. Even though damage to your vision is relatively mild at this stage (in the background), it's a clear warning sign of more-serious damage to come.

In NPDR, high levels of glucose in your bloodstream weaken the walls of the capillaries in your retina. Tiny bulges called microaneurysms protrude from the vessel walls. The microaneurysms may start to leak, oozing blood and fluid into the retina.

Nonproliferative diabetic retinopathy may develop even if your diabetes is

SIGNS OF DIABETIC RETINOPATHY

Among people with diabetic retinopathy, a close examination of the retina generally reveals these characteristic signs:

- **Exudates.** Deposits resembling tiny cream-colored or yellow spots appear around leaking walls of small blood vessels (capillaries) in the retina. Exudates generally don't obscure vision unless they develop in the macula.

- **Cotton-wool spots.** The capillaries that nourish the retina are sometimes blocked off due to chronically high levels of blood glucose. Areas of the retina deprived of nourishment may suffer nerve damage, which appears as white, fluffy wisps on the surface. Tissue damage due to obstructed blood flow is referred to as ischemia.

- **Vitreous hemorrhage.** Blood vessels growing in the retina (neovascularization) are fragile and easily ruptured, especially from the tugs and pulls of a shrinking vitreous. Blood from vessel ruptures and leaking microaneurysms spills into the normally clear vitreous. Minor bleeding may produce a number of dark spots (floaters) in your field of vision. More-severe bleeding can cloud the vitreous, blocking the passage of light to the retina. Bleeding into the vitreous usually doesn't cause permanent vision loss, as treatments are available. The blood eventually clears from the eye, usually within a few months, and your vision returns to its previous clarity, unless the retina has been damaged.

- **Macular edema.** The most frequent cause of vision loss with nonproliferative diabetic retinopathy (NPDR) is from macular edema. Fluid from leaking capillaries accumulates in the macula, causing the tissue to swell. The fluid often forms in cystlike pockets. Symptoms include blurred central vision and objects in your field of vision that appear to have wavy outlines.

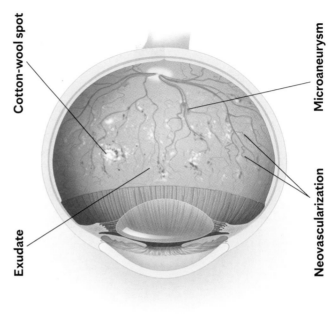

Exudate

Cotton-wool spot

Neovascularization

Microaneurysm

under control. Most often, the symptoms are mild, and they may not affect your ability to see.

Vision problems from NPDR are usually the result of swelling in the macula (macular edema), where fluid and blood leaked from microaneurysms accumulates. Problems also can develop where some capillaries begin to close off, reducing blood flow to the macula (macular ischemia).

On images of the retina, the macula is the reddish patch at the center (see page 15). The macula is essential for central vision. When it can't function properly, your central vision blurs.

Proliferative type

Proliferative diabetic retinopathy (PDR) is a more advanced form of the disease. Many people with very severe NPDR will progress to PDR within a year.

Retinopathy becomes proliferative when many abnormal new blood vessels begin to grow (proliferate) on the retina or the optic nerve. These blood vessels may also grow into the clear vitreous. Because the walls of these blood vessels are extremely fragile and thin, the walls often tear and begin to leak fluid and blood.

The abnormal growth of new blood vessels often follows a widespread closing

NONPROLIFERATIVE DIABETIC RETINOPATHY (NPDR)

Engorged blood vessels, microaneurysms (tiny red dots), bleeding (large red dots) and exudates (yellow spots) are common signs of NPDR. A fluorescein angiogram of the same eye (image at right) shows numerous microaneurysms as intense white dots. The dark spots indicate heavy bleeding and exudates.

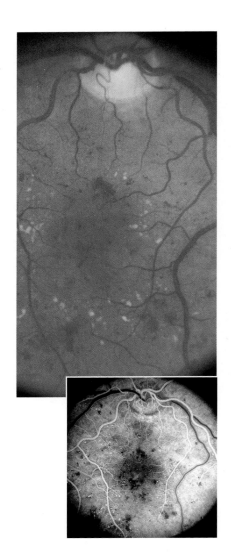

off of capillaries in the eye due to high levels of blood glucose. In an attempt to resupply these areas, the body grows new blood vessels. Unfortunately, these new vessels don't resupply oxygen-starved tissue. Instead, they produce complications affecting both your central and peripheral vision. These complications can include:

Traction retinal detachment

New blood vessels are often accompanied by scar tissue on the retinal surface. As the scar tissue shrinks, it pulls the upper layer away from underlying layers. As the vitreous naturally shrinks due to aging, new blood vessels that have grown into the vitreous begin to tug on the retina. This tension (traction) may cause the retina to detach, forming blank or blurred areas in your visual field.

Neovascular glaucoma

The growth of new blood vessels in the retina may be accompanied by new blood vessels on the iris at the front of the eye. This can increase intraocular pressure, causing a condition known as neovascular glaucoma. Because these changes at the front of the eye stem from problems at

LATE-STAGE PROLIFERATIVE DIABETIC RETINOPATHY (PDR)

In an advanced stage of PDR, abnormal blood vessels grow on the optic nerve and retina and into the vitreous cavity (arrow A). These blood vessels break, causing heavy bleeding (arrow B) and the formation of retinal scar tissue (arrow C).

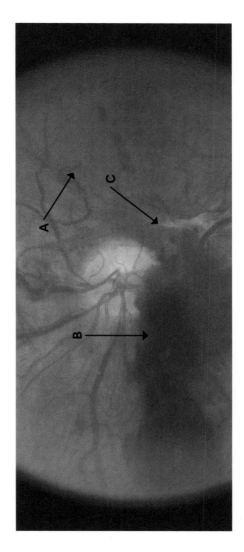

the back of the eye, neovascular glaucoma can be treated with procedures such as panretinal photocoagulation (see page 64). If left untreated, neovascular glaucoma can cause pain, vision loss and, possibly, the loss of an eye.

SIGNS AND SYMPTOMS

In early stages of diabetic retinopathy, most people don't experience signs and symptoms, and changes to vision aren't evident until advanced stages. The best way to detect diabetic retinopathy in its earliest, most treatable stage is to schedule regular eye exams. As diabetic retinopathy progresses to more-advanced stages, visual symptoms may include:

- "Spiders," "cobwebs" or tiny specks floating in your visual field
- Dark streaks or a red film that blocks vision
- General vision loss, but in one eye more than the other
- Blurred vision that may fluctuate
- Dark or empty areas in your vision
- Poor night vision
- Difficulty adjusting from bright light to dim light

RISK FACTORS

As mentioned earlier, the National Eye Institute estimates that more than 2 in 5 Americans with diabetes will experience some form of diabetic retinopathy. You're

BLURRED VISION WITH DIABETES

Blurred vision may be associated with fluctuations in blood glucose levels. Prolonged periods of excessively high blood glucose levels can cause sugar and its byproducts to accumulate in the lens of the eye. This accumulation causes the lens to swell, resulting in nearsightedness, in which distant objects appear blurry. The nearsightedness subsides once blood glucose is brought under control, and the lens can return to its normal thickness.

Blurred vision may also stem from macular swelling (edema), regardless of your blood glucose level. This is of greater concern because untreated macular edema damages central vision. The swelling may fluctuate during the day, making your vision appear to get better or worse.

When new blood vessels form in the vitreous from proliferative diabetic retinopathy (PDR), the vessels may leak, causing dark spots to float in and out of your field of vision. A few days or weeks after the appearance of these floaters, hazy clouds can develop that blur your vision. These are caused by heavy bleeding into the vitreous.

at risk, regardless if you have type 1 or type 2. And your risk increases the longer you have diabetes.

Generally, individuals with type 1 diabetes are at higher risk of retinopathy because they tend to become diabetic at a young age. If you were older than age 30 when you developed diabetes, your risk is lower — although for some, retinopathy can be the first sign of diabetes. Regardless, if you need to take insulin, your risk of retinopathy is increased.

Other risk factors include:
- Poorly controlled diabetes
- High blood pressure
- High blood cholesterol

- Obesity
- Kidney disease
- Pregnancy

SCREENING AND DIAGNOSIS

A common belief among people with diabetes is that as long as they can see well, there's nothing wrong with their eyes. That's a misconception.

Signs and symptoms of diabetic retinopathy can be so subtle that many people are unaware of vision changes. Vision loss often results from people not seeking early medical attention. For this reason, regular eye exams are very important.

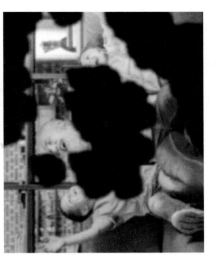

VISION WITH DIABETIC RETINOPATHY

As diabetic retinopathy develops into more-severe stages, your normal vision (shown at left) will become blurred and clouded from bleeding into the vitreous (shown at right). It's possible that some areas of your visual field may be blocked entirely.

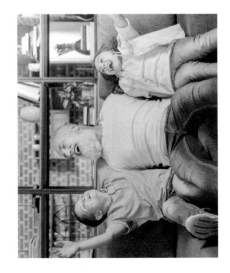

Individuals with diabetes should have a comprehensive dilated eye exam at least once a year. Dilation greatly enlarges your pupil, which gives your eye specialist a better view of your retina with a slit lamp or ophthalmoscope. People with diabetic retinopathy may need more-frequent eye exams.

In addition, if you have diabetes and become pregnant, you should schedule a comprehensive dilated eye exam as soon as possible. Additional eye exams throughout your pregnancy may be recommended.

See an eye doctor promptly if your vision becomes blurry, spotty or hazy. If diabetic retinopathy is detected, your course of treatment will depend on the severity of the condition and whether retinal changes may impair or threaten your vision.

Your eye doctor will likely diagnose diabetic retinopathy — either nonproliferative or proliferative — if an eye exam reveals any of these signs:

- Leaking blood vessels
- Bleeding (hemorrhage) in the retina
- Swollen retina (retinal edema)
- Bulges in blood vessel walls (microaneurysms)
- Fatty deposits (exudates) in the retina
- Nerve fiber damage (cotton-wool spots) in the retina
- Changes in blood vessels, such as closures, beading and loops
- Formation of new blood vessels (neovascularization)
- Bleeding (hemorrhage) into the vitreous
- Formation of scar tissue along with retinal detachment

Your eye examination may include imaging tests such as fluorescein angiography and optical coherence tomography (see pages 50 and 52) to detect leaking blood vessels and swelling of the retina. A newer test called OCT angiography also may be prescribed. This test allows for noninvasive blood flow imaging of the eye. It may be used in addition to or as a replacement for other tests.

TREATMENT

If you're diagnosed with mild nonproliferative diabetic retinopathy (NPDR), you may not require immediate treatment. However, you may have regular eye exams to monitor any ongoing changes to your retina. More-advanced stages of NPDR as well as proliferative diabetic retinopathy (PDR) require prompt treatment, often involving surgery.

The two primary surgical procedures to treat diabetic retinopathy are laser photocoagulation and vitrectomy. Most of the time, these treatments are effective and able to slow or stop the progression of retinopathy for some time.

These procedures aren't a cure. Because diabetes is a systemic disorder that's continually affecting your body, you may still experience retinal damage and vision loss at a later time. You'll need to maintain a regular schedule of eye exams.

Another treatment is medication. Anti-angiogenic drugs that inhibit or stop the growth of abnormal blood vessels (anti-VEGF agents) may be injected into your eye on a regular basis to treat prolifera-tive diabetic retinopathy or slow the progression of nonproliferative retinopa-thy. Medication may also be used to treat swelling of the macula (macular edema). Leakage from the abnormal blood vessels is a primary cause of macular swelling and vitreous hemorrhage, both of which lead to severe vision loss.

Laser photocoagulation

This form of treatment involves the use of a laser to stop the leakage of blood and fluid in the retina, slowing disease progression. There are two types of laser photocoagulation:

Focal photocoagulation

With this treatment, also known as grid macular photocoagulation, a surgeon uses "spot welds" to stop leakage of blood and fluid in the eye. If the leaks are fewer in number, the laser is applied to specific points where the leaks occur — an approach called focal laser treatment. If the leakage is more widespread, burns are applied in a gridlike pattern over a broader area — an approach called grid laser treatment.

The procedure is usually performed in a single session in your doctor's office or at an eye clinic. If you had blurred vision from macular edema before the proce-dure, the treatment might not return your vision to normal. But it's likely to reduce the chance the macular edema and your symptoms may worsen.

Panretinal photocoagulation

This form of laser photocoagulation, also known as scatter laser treatment, is intended to stop new blood vessel growth. During the procedure, retinal areas away from the macula are treated with scattered laser burns. The burns cause the abnormal new blood vessels to shrink and scar.

The treatment usually involves two or more sessions. Your vision may be blurry for about a day after the procedure. Some loss of peripheral vision or night vision after the procedure is possible.

Your eye doctor may recommend photo-coagulation if you have:

- Swelling (edema) of the retina that involves the macula
- A severe stage of nonproliferative diabetic retinopathy and are unable to return for frequent follow-up visits
- Proliferative diabetic retinopathy
- Neovascular glaucoma

Before the procedure gets underway, your pupil is dilated and anesthetic drops are used to numb the eye. In certain cases, the eye is numbed com-pletely with an injection. With your head resting in front of a slit lamp, a special lens is placed on your cornea to help focus the laser light onto sections of the retina to be treated. Fluorescein angio-grams taken beforehand may be used to indicate where the burns should be placed.

During the procedure, a high-energy laser beam burns small, pinpoint areas of the

PANRETINAL PHOTOCOAGULATION

Doctors often treat proliferative diabetic retinopathy (PDR), in which many new blood vessels are forming, with panretinal photocoagulation, also known as scatter laser treatment. With this technique, multiple laser burns hit the entire retina except for the macula. The treatment causes the abnormal vessels to shrink and disappear over a wide area, reducing the chance of vitreous bleeding and traction retinal detachment.

Panretinal photocoagulation may be performed in one or more sessions. You may or may not notice some loss of side (peripheral) vision afterward. The procedure is a trade-off. Some of your side vision may be diminished to save as much of your central vision as possible. You may also notice difficulties with your night vision.

Panretinal photocoagulation alone doesn't always stop vision loss from diabetic retinopathy, even with repeated treatments. It may need to be combined with other forms of treatment, including injections of medication into the eye or surgery.

This treatment covers most of the retina outside the macula. The mass of yellow spots on the image below indicates where laser burns were applied to close off blood vessels and stop the leaking.

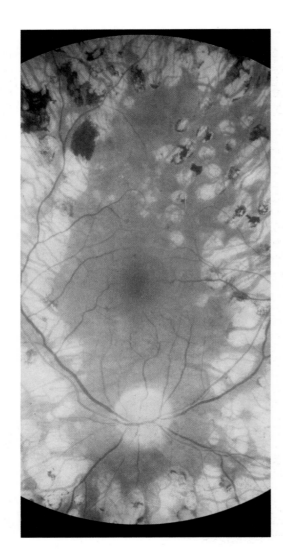

retina. You may see bright flashes from the high-energy bursts. The burns seal off the vessels and stop the leakage of fluid and blood (see the opposite page).

After the treatment, your vision may be blurry for about a day. Small spots resulting from laser burns may appear in your visual field. You should be able to return home, but you won't be able to drive, so make sure to arrange for someone drive you. You may have some eye pain or a headache and be sensitive to light. An eye patch and over-the-counter pain relievers should help to ease any discomfort.

Even when laser surgery is successful at sealing the leaks, new blood vessels may continue to grow and new leakage may occur. For this reason, you'll need follow-up visits and, if necessary, additional laser treatments.

Vitrectomy

Sometimes, blood that has leaked (hemorrhaged) from abnormal blood vessels into the vitreous will gradually clear up on its own. But if the bleeding is heavy and it doesn't clear, the clouded vitreous will block the passage of light to your retina and interfere with your vision.

A surgical procedure known as a vitrectomy may be required to remove the blockage. Removal of the blood enables your eye specialist to better monitor your diabetic retinopathy and any swelling (macular edema) and to treat the conditions when needed.

Vitrectomy is performed using a microscope suspended over the eye that allows the surgeon to see the eye's interior in much greater detail. A light probe also illuminates the eye to help the surgeon see better. Several delicate instruments are inserted through small incisions made in the eye to remove the blood-filled vitreous. The surgeon uses a vitreous cutter to cut the tissue, which is suctioned out. To maintain the shape and internal pressure of the eye, an infusion tube injects a balanced salt solution to replace the tissue being removed. Removal of the blood-filled vitreous generally reestablishes clear vision.

A vitrectomy may also be performed to remove scar tissue from the retina. This action reduces the steady force (traction) pulling the retina away from underlying layers, allowing a detached retina to settle back and flatten out. A surgeon may decide not to operate on a retina detached by scar tissue if the detachment is located away from the macula and doesn't appear to be getting worse.

Gas or silicone oil is usually put in the internal cavity in place of the removed portion of the vitreous. This creates a gentle pressure that helps keep the retina attached to the back of the eye. The gas dissolves in about three to eight weeks. The silicone oil may be removed from the eye several months later; however, in the most severe cases, it may be kept in. When the oil is removed, the cavity refills with natural fluids.

Local or general anesthesia may be used during a vitrectomy. Your eye will likely

An external view (bottom image) shows two instruments inserted into the eyeball: a vitreous cutter (A) and a light probe (B). Although the surgeon views the procedure through a surgical microscope, a specially designed lens held directly over the eye is also required (C). An interior view of the procedure (image at right) shows the cutter removing scar tissue (D) illuminated by the light probe (E). A saline solution (F) is added to help maintain the shape of the eyeball.

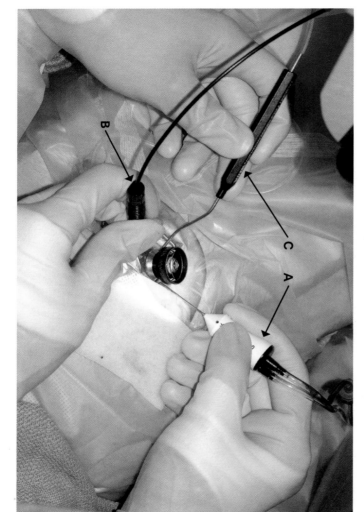

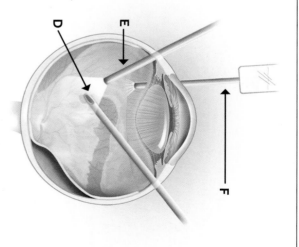

be red, swollen and sensitive to light afterward. For a short time, you'll need to wear an eye patch and apply medicated eye drops to assist in healing.

Panretinal photocoagulation may also be performed during a vitrectomy to prevent the renewed growth of abnormal blood vessels.

Full recovery from the procedure may take weeks. When a vitrectomy is performed in case of massive bleeding, some blood may remain in the vitreous. Sometimes, fresh bleeding may occur. As the blood gradually dissipates, your sight should return to its former clarity.

How well you'll see after surgery depends on the health of your retina. If the retina and macula have good blood flow and appear healthy, your vision may improve.

If there isn't a healthy blood supply to the retina or there's irreparable damage to the retina, the procedure may not improve your vision, but it may help to stabilize it. Complications from surgery, recurring bleeding from torn blood vessels or the development of neovascular glaucoma also can keep vision from improving.

Intravitreal injections

Another form of treatment for diabetic retinopathy and macular edema is to inject medication into the eye's vitreous. There are currently several medications approved by the Food and Drug Administration (FDA) for this purpose. They fall into two categories:

- Medications that inhibit vascular endothelial growth factor (VEGF)

ANTI-VEGF THERAPY

Below is an optical coherence tomography (OCT) scan. The image on the left shows a swollen macula from fluid accumulation in a cystlike pocket (arrow). Following treatment with bevacizumab (Avastin), a later scan of the same eye (right) reveals that the edema has diminished and the macula has returned to normal contours.

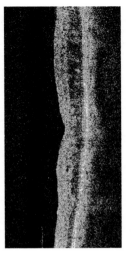
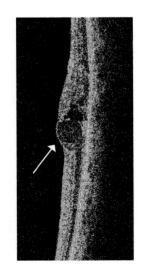

- Steroid medications that reduce inflammation

Medications known as VEGF inhibitors, such as bevacizumab (Avastin), ranibizumab (Lucentis) and aflibercept (Eylea), help stop the growth of new blood vessels by blocking the effects of growth signals the body sends to generate new blood vessels. Your doctor may recommend these medications, also known as anti-VEGF therapy, as a stand-alone treatment or in combination with another treatment.

Swelling in the macula (macular edema) is the result of high levels of VEGF and high levels of inflammation in the vitreous cavity. Anti-VEGF agents are among the medications used to treat diabetic macular edema, as well as the steroid medications dexamethasone (Ozurdex) and fluocinolone (Iluvien). The steroid drugs come in the form of tiny implants that are injected into the eye's vitreous. In the eye, they slowly release medication over time without the need for regular injections.

With anti-VEGF agents, injections are usually given monthly. As the eye responds, they may be given every two months, then less often. Steroid implant injections can last three to six months (dexamethasone) or two to three years (fluocinolone).

Before injection, the eye is numbed with eye drops, and the surface of the eye is sterilized. The most common side effect of these injections is a scratchy sensation on the surface of the eye that lasts about a day. Rarely, a serious eye infection can

occur (endophthalmitis) that may require surgery to treat the infection.

In addition to intravitreal injections, other new treatments also are being studied to treat macular edema and diabetic retinopathy.

SELF-CARE

There are a variety of steps that you can take to help keep your diabetes under control and effectively slow the progression of diabetic retinopathy.

Control your blood glucose

Tight control of your blood sugar (glucose) slows the onset and progression of retinal damage and lessens the need for surgery. Tight control means keeping your blood glucose levels as close to normal as possible.

Ideally, this means glucose levels between 80 and 130 milligrams of sugar per deciliter of blood (mg/dL) before meals and less than 180 mg/dL two hours after the start of a meal. Your blood sugar targets may be different depending on your age, additional health issues and other factors. Talk to your medical provider about what targets are best for you.

Another measure of good control is your glycated hemoglobin level. The glycated hemoglobin test, called the hemoglobin A1C test, measures how well you've controlled your blood glucose level over the previous two to three months. The

A1C goal for most adults with diabetes is around 7% or less, but your goal may be different depending on other factors.

Tight control isn't possible for everyone, including some older adults, young children and people with cardiovascular disease. Talk to your medical provider or diabetes educator about a management plan that's best suited to your lifestyle and your personal goals. A management plan frequently involves:

• Taking regular doses of insulin or other medications
• Monitoring blood glucose levels
• Following a healthy-eating plan
• Getting regular exercise
• Maintaining a healthy weight

Remember that poorly controlled blood glucose is often a root cause for abnormal blood vessel leakage in your retina. And it may be a while before the benefits of lowering your blood glucose level are fully realized. Also keep in mind that improved control reduces but doesn't totally eliminate your risk of developing retinopathy.

Be alert for vision changes

In addition to having yearly eye exams, be alert for any sudden changes in your vision. Have your eyes checked as soon as possible if you experience changes that:

• Last more than a few days
• Aren't associated with changes in blood glucose levels
• Appear to be blurry, spotty or hazy
• Include eye pain, redness, floaters or light flashes

Reduce your blood pressure

High blood pressure is also a major risk factor for diabetic retinopathy. Elevated blood pressure that goes untreated may damage tiny capillaries, which can trigger the formation of abnormal new blood vessels on the retina. So, keeping your blood pressure under control can be a powerful preventive measure.

If you have diabetic retinopathy, studies indicate that reducing your blood pressure may help slow progression of your retinopathy. To reduce your blood pressure, you'll need to make certain lifestyle changes and you may need medication.

Stop smoking

Smoking is especially harmful for people with diabetes and high blood pressure because tobacco use can slow or block blood circulation.

Limit alcohol

Consuming more than moderate amounts of alcohol can increase your blood pressure, affect your blood sugar levels and interfere with medications you're taking.

Maintain a healthy weight

Your weight, blood pressure and blood glucose tend to go hand in hand. When your weight increases, so do your blood pressure and blood glucose levels. Being overweight also is a key risk factor for

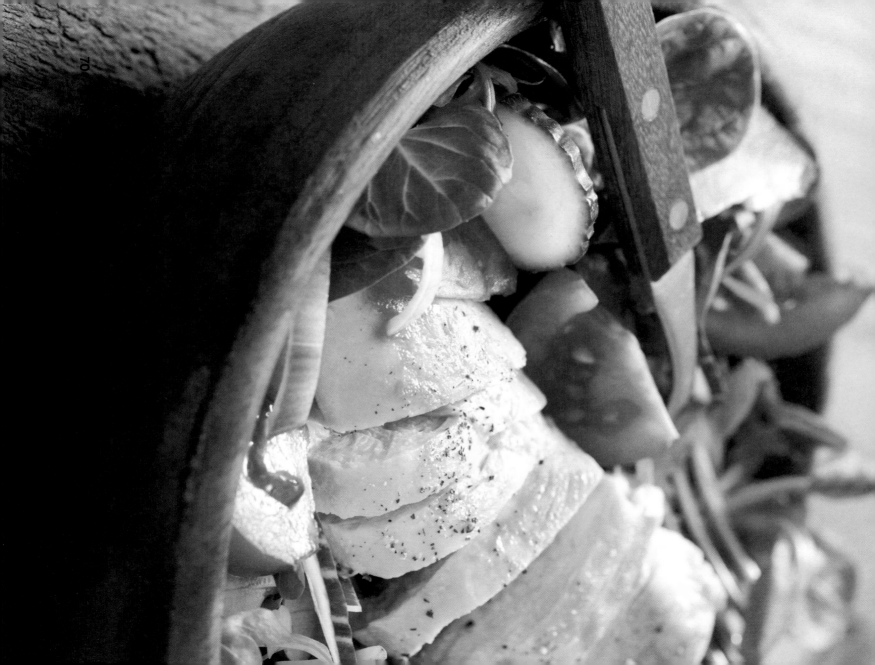

diabetes. As Americans become increasingly overweight, controlling weight has become a major challenge in preventing and treating high blood pressure and diabetes.

The best way to control your weight is with a healthy diet and regular exercise. Find an eating plan that emphasizes vegetables, fruits, whole grains, low-fat dairy, fish and lean meats, and healthy fats to help you lose weight.

Exercise

Regular physical activity helps control diabetes by reducing the level of blood sugar (glucose) in your bloodstream. Physical activity is also a key factor for managing many other chronic conditions, including high blood pressure. Aim for at least 30 minutes of aerobic activity most days of the week. Bouts of activity can be as brief as 10 minutes, three times a day. If you haven't been active in a while, start slowly and build up gradually.

Control stress

Stress can cause wide swings in blood pressure and blood glucose levels. Stress may also affect your ability to control your diabetes. For example, stress may leave you too busy or preoccupied to exercise or eat healthy or to socialize with friends and family. Don't hesitate to seek help from a counselor, therapist or support group. Relaxation techniques such as meditation and deep breathing also may be helpful.

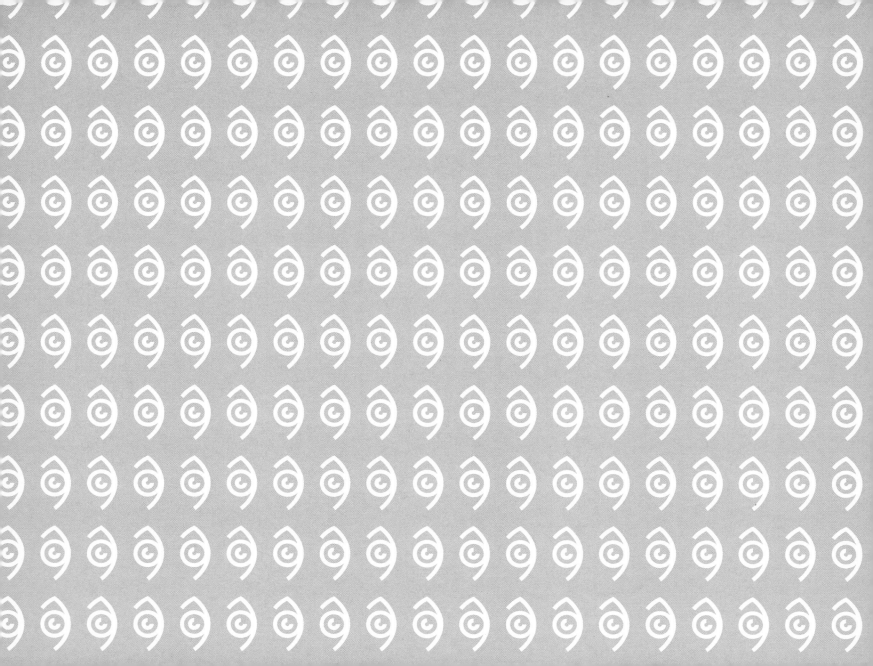

4

Other retinal and optic nerve disorders

Previous chapters looked at major diseases that damage the eye's retina, specifically age-related macular degeneration (AMD) and diabetic retinopathy. This chapter focuses on other conditions that can affect the retina and optic nerve, including retinal detachment.

As mentioned earlier, the retina is a thin layer of tissue at the back of the eye that converts light into electric signals. Attached to the back of the retina is the optic nerve, a bundle of nerve fibers along which electric signals travel back and forth between the eye and the brain.

Over time, changes can occur to the retina and optic nerve that affect almost everyone's vision at some point. These conditions often are harmless. However, other, less common changes may develop

that can lead to vision loss, if the conditions are left untreated.

FLOATERS AND FLASHES

The large internal cavity of your eye is filled with a clear, jellylike substance called the vitreous humor or, simply, the vitreous. Eye floaters are small bits of debris floating in the vitreous.

Floaters may appear as tiny spots, hairs or bits of string that randomly dart in and out of your field of vision. Floaters are most noticeable in bright light: for example, a sunny day in winter or a well-lit room with white walls.

Floaters are due to age-related changes to the vitreous. Over time, the consistency of the vitreous changes and it partially liquefies, a process causing it to shrink and pull away from the interior surface of the eye. This is called posterior vitreous detachment (PVD), or vitreous collapse.

Other factors that can lead to vitreous detachment include nearsightedness, eye trauma, inflammation, diseases such as diabetic retinopathy and complications of cataract surgery.

Vitreous collapse itself doesn't cause vision loss and no treatment may be necessary. But shrinking does cause the vitreous to become fibrous and stringy. When floaters appear in your visual field, what you're often seeing are the shadows these strings cast on the retina. Although bothersome, floaters generally don't pose a serious problem.

FLOATERS

Tiny pieces of debris floating in the vitreous block some of the light passing through the eye's interior, casting shadows on the retina that appear as dark specks in your vision.

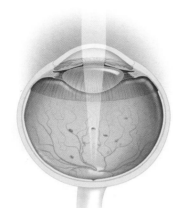

Along with floaters, you may see flashes of sparkling lights in your side (peripheral) vision when your eyes are closed or if you're in a darkened room. This phenomenon generally is brief, lasting only a few seconds.

The flashes occur because some of the fibers in the vitreous are still attached to the retina and, as the vitreous sags, pull on the retinal surface. The flashes appear in your side vision because the fibers tend to be more firmly attached to the retina around its periphery.

Floaters generally increase in number gradually with age. In rare instances, the number and size of the floaters may interfere with your central vision. In such cases, a doctor may recommend surgical removal of the floating debris with a procedure called vitrectomy. However, this surgery carries risks, including bleeding and retinal tears.

There may be times when floaters are a much greater concern. See your eye doctor immediately if you notice a sudden onset or significant increase in floaters — especially if they're accompanied by sparkling lights or hazy vision. These changes signal a potentially serious eye disorder, such as a retinal tear or retinal detachment.

MACULAR PUCKER

The sagging and tugging of the vitreous on the retina can cause microscopic damage to the retinal surface. As part of the healing process, scar tissue may form around the damaged areas. Typically, the scar tissue begins to shrink, causing the retina to wrinkle or pucker.

A small amount of scar tissue generally has little effect on vision. But when enough scar tissue builds up on the macula, forming a prominent pucker, your vision may become blurred or distorted. You may have difficulty seeing fine detail. Part of your central vision may become clouded.

The symptoms of a macular pucker — blurriness and distortion — are often mild and require no treatment. People simply adjust to the change. Vision usually stabilizes after the initial change and doesn't progressively worsen. Usually just one eye is affected, but puckers may occur in both eyes. A pucker generally doesn't cause a tear or hole to form on the macular surface.

If the symptoms become more severe, surgery may be necessary to remove the scar tissue.

RETINAL TEAR AND MACULAR HOLE

If the pull of a sagging vitreous is strong enough, the retina may tear, forming a small, jagged flap on its surface. Most tears occur along the periphery of the retina, where firmly attached fibers in the vitreous can't separate without hard tugging.

Retinal tears and holes are associated with aging and usually occur in people older than age 60. The tears and holes are usually caused by a shrinking vitreous, but retinal holes may also develop where the retina has simply become thin. Other causes of retinal tears and holes include nearsightedness and eye trauma.

If a hole forms in the macula instead of along the periphery, the consequences are more noticeable to your central vision. In early stages, there may be blurred vision — comparable to the vision changes from a macular pucker. However, the two conditions are very different.

Some small retinal holes generally require no treatment and seal themselves as the tissue heals. In some cases, fluid from the vitreous seeps through the tear and pools under the surface of the retina, causing surrounding sections to detach from the underlying layer. This can lead to severe vision loss.

Treating retinal tears

If the retina hasn't already detached from the underlying layer of tissue surrounding the tear, your surgeon may suggest one of two procedures to treat it. With either procedure, healing typically takes between 10 and 14 days, during which time you would need to refrain from vigorous activity.

Photocoagulation

In this procedure, a surgeon directs a laser beam to make burns around the retinal tear. The burns cause scarring, which usually "welds" the retina to the

underlying tissue. This procedure requires no surgical incision and it causes
less irritation to the eye than does
cryopexy.

Cryopexy

In this procedure, a surgeon uses intense
cold to freeze tissue around the retinal
tear instead of applying heat from a laser.
After a local anesthetic has numbed your
eye, a freezing probe is applied to the
outer surface of the eye directly over the
tear. The freezing produces inflammation
that causes scarring, welding the retina to

the underlying tissue, much as with
photocoagulation.

Cryopexy is an alternative treatment in
cases when the tear is more difficult to
reach with a laser, generally along the
retinal periphery. Your eye may be red
and swollen for some time after the
procedure.

RETINAL DETACHMENT

Retinal detachment is a medical emergency, and timing is critical when it
comes to treating the condition. Unless

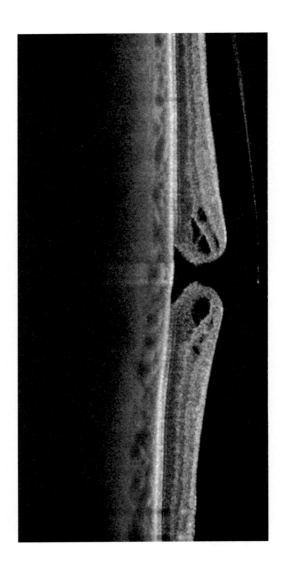

MACULAR HOLE

A cross section of the retina on this optical coherence tomography scan
reveals a large hole in the macula, which can blur vision and cause visual
distortions.

the detached retina can be surgically reattached promptly, this condition causes permanent vision loss or blindness in the affected eye.

Retinal detachment occurs when fluid leaking through a tear or break causes part of the retina to peel away from underlying layers, such as the retinal pigment epithelium and choroid. As liquid collects under the retina from continued leakage, the detachment expands, similar to wallpaper slowly peeling off a wall. Areas where the retina is detached can no longer function, and vision progressively blurs.

TYPES OF RETINAL DETACHMENT

Following are names used to describe various types of retinal detachments.

Rhegmatogenous

This type of retinal detachment is the most common. Rhegmatogenous detachments are caused by a hole or tear in the retina that allows fluid to pass through and collect underneath the retina, pulling the retina away from underlying tissues. The areas where the retina detaches lose their blood supply and stop working, causing you to lose vision.

The most common cause of rhegmatogenous detachment is aging. With age, the eye's vitreous may change in consistency and shrink. Normally, the vitreous separates from the surface of the retina without any complications. But sometimes as the vitreous separates or peels off the retina, it may tug on the retina with enough force to create a retinal tear. Left untreated, the liquid vitreous can pass through the tear into the space behind the retina, causing the retina to become detached.

Tractional

This type of detachment can occur when scar tissue grows on the retina's surface, causing the retina to pull away from the back of the eye. Tractional detachment is typically seen in people who have poorly controlled diabetes or other conditions.

Exudative

In this type of detachment, fluid accumulates beneath the retina, but there are no holes or tears in the retina. Another name for this type of detachment is serous retinal detachment. Exudative detachment can be caused by age-related macular degeneration, injury to the eye, tumors or inflammatory disorders.

Not all tears and holes in the retina lead to retinal detachment. Sometimes the retinal tissue surrounding these defects remains relatively well attached. But more often, the leakage of fluid from the vitreous causes separation.

Detachment that goes undetected and untreated can eventually involve the entire retina. Typically, scar tissue forms on the surface and the retina becomes stiff. This is known as proliferative vitreoretinopathy. At this stage, even if extensive surgery is performed, it's unlikely that you'll regain the vision that you had before the detachment occurred.

Other, less common causes of retinal detachment include traction from a buildup of scar tissue on the retinal surface. This can occur in people with diabetes. Sometimes, retinal detachment may occur without a tear on the retina. This is known as serous retinal detachment. The condition can stem from the leakage of fluid under the retina due to trauma, a tumor or an inflammatory condition.

Signs and symptoms

Retinal detachment is generally painless, but warning signs typically appear before the detachment occurs. Warning signs may include one or more of the following events:

• The sudden appearance of many new floaters; when your retina tears, pigment may be released into the vitreous, or small blood vessels may break and leak blood that seeps into the vitreous

• Sudden bright flashes of light in the affected eye

• What resembles a shadow or curtain falling over part of your visual field

• Sudden blurriness in your vision; because most tears occur along the periphery of the retina, the blurring may first become noticeable in your peripheral vision

If you experience any of these signs or symptoms, seek immediate care from an ophthalmologist. Although floaters or flashes typically don't indicate a serious problem, if they happen to be caused by retinal detachment, prompt treatment is critical to preserve your vision.

Unfortunately, many people don't heed the urgency of the warning signs. They tend to delay seeing an eye specialist in the hope that the symptoms disappear. On some occasions, the symptoms do diminish — but then a sudden, drastic loss of vision may occur over the following days or weeks, caused by untreated, advanced retinal detachment.

Retinal detachment can't always be successfully repaired with surgery, and vision loss may become permanent. That's why it's important to see your eye doctor as soon as you notice that something isn't right with your vision.

Risk factors

Your risk of developing a detached retina generally increases with age, simply because of changes to the vitreous as you grow older. A detached retina is more common among men than women. You're also at greater risk if any of these factors apply:

- Previous retinal detachment in one eye
- Family history of retinal detachment
- Extreme nearsightedness
- Previous eye surgery, such as cataract removal
- Previous severe eye injury or eye trauma

- Weak areas along the periphery of your retina

An eye doctor will likely examine your eye with an ophthalmoscope, an instrument that provides a highly detailed view of the retina to detect any tears, holes or detachments. Additional examinations or tests also may be performed.

RETINAL DETACHMENT

A section of the retina that has pulled away from the back wall of the eye appears darker and folded (upper right) on this color photograph. Most detachments occur in the upper part of the eyeball due to the effects of gravity on the sagging vitreous (see inset).

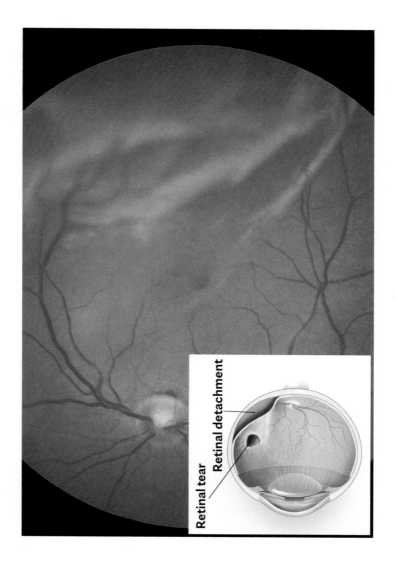

Retinal tear

Retinal detachment

Surgery is the only effective therapy for a retinal detachment. If a tear or hole on the retina can be treated before detachment begins, or if a detachment is treated before the macula is affected, you'll likely retain much of your vision. It's best if the surgery can be performed within days of a diagnosis.

Different surgical procedures may be used to repair a detached retina. Pneumatic retinopexy and scleral buckling are performed with cryopexy (see page 83). Vitrectomy may be necessary to clear a massive hemorrhage in the vitreous or to remove scar tissue (see page 66).

Treatment goals are to reseal the tear and stop fluid from collecting underneath the retina, reduce the tug of a shrinking vitreous on the retina, and reattach the loosened portion of the retina. The severity and complexity of the detachment will determine which treatment your surgeon recommends.

Pneumatic retinopexy

Pneumatic retinopexy is used for an uncomplicated detachment when the tear is located in the upper half of the retina. The procedure is usually done on an outpatient basis under local anesthesia.

A surgeon uses cold (cryopexy) to seal the tear and then withdraws fluid from the anterior chamber to soften the eye. Next, a gas bubble is injected into the vitreous. The gas bubble expands, pushing against

PNEUMATIC RETINOPEXY

After sealing a retinal tear with cryopexy, a gas bubble is injected into the vitreous. The bubble applies gentle pressure, helping a detached section of the retina to reattach to the eyeball. The eye gradually absorbs the gas bubble over several weeks.

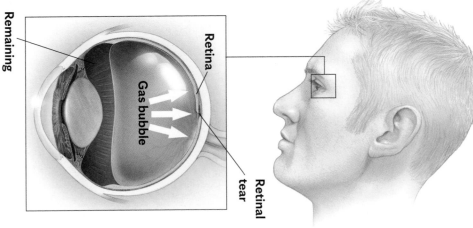

Retina

Gas bubble

Retinal tear

Remaining fluid in eye

can usually be repaired with scleral buckling or vitrectomy.

Scleral buckling

Slightly reducing the physical circumference of the eye can help reattach the retina and relieve tension caused by a shrinking vitreous. Called scleral buckling, this procedure is usually performed in an operating room under local or general anesthesia and often on an outpatient basis.

First, a surgeon treats the retinal tear with cryopexy. Then he or she indents (buckles) the sclera immediately over the affected area by pressing on the eyeball with silicone material — either a soft sponge or a solid piece.

Gentle external pressure provided by the buckle helps close the separation between the retina and underlying layers. It also promotes healing. By reducing the size of the eyeball, the buckle eases some of the tugging by the vitreous, helping prevent further retinal tears.

For a single tear with no other problems than detachment, the buckle may be placed directly over the detached area. For multiple tears or an extensive detachment, the surgeon may use a scleral buckle that encircles the eyeball.

The buckle is stitched to the outer surface of the sclera. Before tying the sutures that hold the buckle in place, the surgeon may make a tiny cut in the sclera to drain fluid that has collected under the detached retina. With no more fluid moving through the tear, the retina reattaches itself to the back of the eye. Sometimes, laser photocoagulation can be used as well as, or instead of, cryopexy.

After surgery, you may have to hold your head in a certain position for several days to keep the bubble in place. It takes several weeks for it to disappear completely. Until the gas is gone, you should avoid lying or sleeping on your back to keep the bubble away from your lens, thereby reducing the risk of cataract formation or a sudden increase of pressure in your eye.

During recovery, you can't travel by airplane or be at a high altitude because a sudden drop in pressure would cause the gas bubble to expand rapidly, resulting in dangerously high pressure in your eye. Your surgeon can advise you on when the danger has passed.

The success of pneumatic retinopexy depends on many factors, and among carefully selected individuals, can prevent the need for incisional surgery.

Complications may include:
• Recurring retinal detachment
• Excessive scar tissue formation
• Cataracts
• Glaucoma (due to an increase in pressure from the gas bubble)
• Gas collecting under the retina
• Infection

These complications are rare, but if they do occur and go untreated they can cause severe vision loss. Recurring detachments the detached retina. The buckle remains in place for the rest of your life.

Scleral buckling is often successful, but reattaching the retina doesn't guarantee that you'll have normal vision. How well you see after the procedure depends in part on how much of the retina was detached and for how long it was de-tached.

Your sight isn't likely to return to normal if the macula was detached at some point. Even if the macula was unaffected and scleral buckling successfully repairs a retinal detachment, you may lose some vision over the long term due to wrinkling or puckering of the macula. If the proce-

dure fails the first time, the surgeon may reattach the retina with additional operations. Additional surgery increases the rate of success.

Sometimes, after scleral buckling, the retina fails to firmly reattach. This may be due to existing scar tissue on the retinal surface. But scar tissue can also form after the procedure, which may cause the retina to separate after having been reattached. If this happens, it's usually within the first couple of months after surgery. More surgery may become necessary to remove the scar tissue.

Complications from scleral buckling occur infrequently but may result in the

BLEEDING IN THE VITREOUS

When blood spills into the vitreous cavity from torn blood vessels around a retinal tear, it's called a vitreous hemorrhage. Diagnosing and treating retinal detachment in the presence of a vitreous hemorrhage can be difficult because blood clouds the vitreous and prevents the surgeon from getting a clear view of the retina. Ultrasonography may be used to locate the retinal tear and assess the damage.

Ultrasonography is an imaging test that sends sound waves through the clouded vitreous to bounce off the retina. The returning sound waves are collected in a digital image that allows the doctor to determine the condition of the retina and other structures inside the eye. If a retinal detachment is found, a vitrectomy may be required to remove blood from the vitreous before the surgeon can repair the retina.

In this circumstance you're at high risk of developing scar tissue in the vitreous and on the retina, a condition called proliferative vitreoretinopathy. The condition occurs when scar tissue folds or puckers the retina, preventing it from being reattached by standard surgical means.

loss of some or all vision in the eye or, in rare instances, the loss of the eye. Complications may include:

- Bleeding under the retina or into the vitreous cavity. This may occur inadvertently while fluid beneath the retina is being drained or when stitching punctures the sclera.
- Increased pressure inside the eye. This may be due to a swelling of the choroid and narrowing of the angle in the anterior chamber.
- Double vision (diplopia). This common side effect occurs when a buckle passes underneath an eye muscle. The condition is usually temporary and may require corrective lenses. Occasionally, surgery is needed to remove the buckle or reposition the muscle.

Vitrectomy

Sometimes, extensive bleeding or inflammation clouds the vitreous, blocking the surgeon's view of the retina. Other times, scar tissue makes it impossible to repair a retinal detachment. In these situations, a procedure called vitrectomy may be required to remove the clouded vitreous.

During a vitrectomy, a surgeon removes the vitreous along with any tissue that is tugging on the retina. Air, gas or silicone oil is then injected into the vitreous space to replace the fluid removed and help flatten the retina. Scleral buckling may be included with the procedure to correct a retinal detachment.

Eventually the air, gas or liquid will be absorbed, and the vitreous space will refill with body fluid. If silicone oil was used, it may be surgically removed months later.

ENCIRCLING SCLERAL BUCKLE

Silicone material stitched to the outside of the eye indents or "buckles" the sclera, making the eyeball smaller. A smaller circumference assists the healing process by pushing the choroid against the detached retina. It also reduces the amount of traction placed on the retina by a shrinking vitreous.

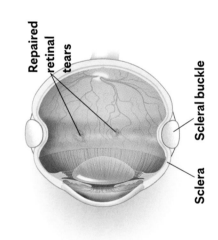

Repaired retinal tears

Sclera   **Scleral buckle**

After surgery

Expect your eye to be red, swollen, watery and slightly sore for up to a month after any of the surgical procedures just described. Wearing an eye patch may provide temporary relief.

Your surgeon may prescribe a combination of anti-inflammatory, antibacterial or

Other retinal and optic nerve disorders   83

dilating eye drops to help the healing process. Severe pain is unlikely but should it occur, contact your surgeon immediately for treatment.

It'll take about 8 to 10 weeks for your eye to heal fully. You should avoid all strenuous activities during this time. As your vision stabilizes, your ophthalmologist can determine whether you'll need corrective lenses or adjustments to an existing prescription. Your vision may take many months to improve after surgery to repair a complicated retinal detachment. Some people never recover all of their lost vision.

RETINAL BLOOD VESSEL BLOCKAGE

Intricate networks of arteries and veins support the retina. The blood vessels are close together, sometimes crossing over and intertwining with each other. The networks connect to major blood vessels — the central retinal artery and the central retinal vein — that enter the eye through the optic nerve.

Sometimes, these arteries and veins can become blocked, a condition known as retinal vessel occlusion. The condition is common in older adults and can result in reduced vision or vision loss.

Various factors can obstruct a blood vessel, such as a blood clot, the accumulation of fatty deposits (plaques) in the vessel, the collapse of a vessel wall or compression of a wall from outside pressure. When a retinal artery is obstructed, oxygen-rich blood is unable to nourish the retina. When a retinal vein is obstructed, the blood backs up, causing the retina to swell.

The location of the blockage, the presence of swelling and how much time elapses before treatment are key factors. Several conditions can result from blockage of blood vessels in the retina.

Branch retinal vein occlusion (BRVO)

Blockage causes blood to back up in the capillaries and pressure to build in the retina. The pressure leads to bleeding from the capillaries and swelling (edema) in the macula, blurring vision or causing "blind spots." BRVO is one of the most common retinal circulatory disorders.

Macular swelling may be treated with anti-angiogenic injections (see page 42), or focal (grid macular) photocoagulation (see page 63).

A complication of BRVO is the growth of new blood vessels on the optic nerve, retina or iris. Left untreated, these vessels may hemorrhage in the vitreous. Vessel growth on the iris may cause neovascular glaucoma and irreversible loss of vision. Panretinal laser treatment (see page 63), possibly combined with anti-angiogenic eye injections, may be used to halt the new vessel growth.

Central retinal vein occlusion (CRVO)

Blockage may occur in the large retinal vein, which collects blood passing through the capillaries. CRVO causes branch veins to engorge and the retina surrounding the optic nerve to swell.

Vision loss may be mild to severe. As with BRVO, vision loss occurs from poor blood supply to the retina and leakage from capillaries, causing macular edema. Unlike BRVO, grid laser photocoagulation isn't effective. The condition must be treated with steroid or anti-angiogenic injections.

New blood vessel growth on the optic nerve, retina or iris may also occur with CRVO and may be treated with the panretinal laser procedure, sometimes combined with anti-angiogenic eye injections.

RETINAL VEIN OCCLUSION

Blockage of the retinal veins causes a backup of blood and swelling in the macula, blurring vision and creating blind spots in your visual field.

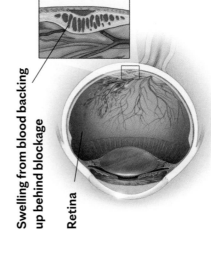

Swelling from blood backing up behind blockage

Retina

Branch retinal artery occlusion (BRAO)

Blockage may occur in a small branch artery, limiting blood supply to the retina. The blockage is often the result of a blood clot or abnormal particle (embolus) that lodges in the vessel. An early indication of the condition is usually partial vision loss — sometimes central vision — that happens abruptly. Currently, there's no proven treatment to regain loss of vision.

The most common cause of BRAO is an embolus. Other causes include inflammation of the blood vessels (vasculitis) or the eye (uveitis) and clotting abnormalities. Risk factors include high blood pressure, high cholesterol, abnormal clotting, diabetes, coronary artery disease and narrowing of the carotid artery.

Central retinal artery occlusion (CRAO)

CRAO is a medical emergency. In this condition, blockage of the main retinal artery significantly obstructs blood flow to the retina. The condition may be referred to as a "stroke" of the eye and generally results in sudden, profound vision loss. Causes and risk factors are similar to those of BRAO.

If you experience sudden vision loss in an eye, go to an emergency department or see an eye specialist immediately. CRAO increases the risk of systemic stroke.

There currently is no proven treatment for CRAO. Experimental treatments are aimed at dislodging the obstruction from the blood vessel. Chances of improved vision are best if treatment occurs less than 24 hours from symptom onset.

DISORDERS OF THE OPTIC NERVE

The optic nerve is the pathway that allows the eye to communicate with the brain. It's analogous to a high-speed fiber-optic cable linking homes with television and internet service. Problems with the optic nerve may interfere with the transmission of electrical impulses produced by the retina and interpreted by the brain, resulting in vision loss.

Optic neuritis

Optic neuritis is an inflammation of the optic nerve. Optic neuritis is believed to develop when the body's immune system

CENTRAL RETINAL ARTERY OCCLUSION

The pale retina on this color photograph is a result of blockage in the central retinal artery that prevents sufficient blood flow to the eye.

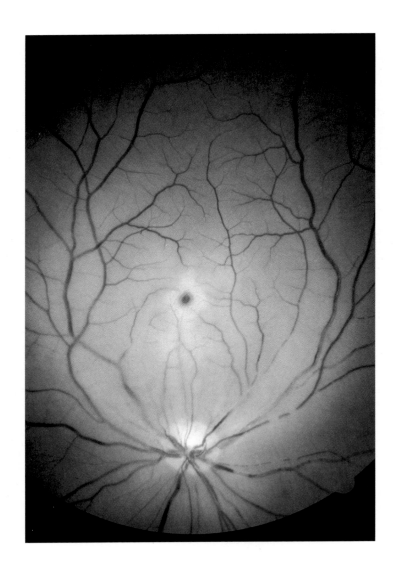

mistakenly targets a substance covering the optic nerve called myelin; however, the exact cause of this condition is unknown. Certain autoimmune diseases, such as multiple sclerosis, are often associated with the disease.

When the condition affects only the optic disk, where the optic nerve is attached to the eye, it's known as papillitis. When the inflammation occurs in the portion of the optic nerve behind the eye, it's known as retrobulbar neuritis.

When the optic nerve swells due to the inflammation, it blocks signals to the brain. The result is a gradual or sudden loss of vision, usually in one eye, but it may occur in both. Most people experience eye pain that's worse with eye movement. In the case of papillitis, vision loss is the only symptom.

Optic neuritis usually gets better on its own. In some cases, steroid medications are prescribed to help reduce inflammation. Most people regain close to normal vision within a year after an episode.

If you have optic neuritis, magnetic resonance imaging (MRI) may be performed to determine your risk of multiple sclerosis (MS). If you appear to be at high risk of MS, you may benefit from treatment with drugs that can help prevent it.

Papilledema

Papilledema is a swelling of the optic disk caused by an elevated pressure within the skull.

The abnormally high pressure may be caused by a tumor, abscess, hemorrhage or infection in the brain.

Vision usually isn't affected in early stages of papilledema. As the condition progresses, symptoms such as blurred vision may occur briefly, then disappear. Treatment will depend on the cause — for example, surgery to remove a tumor or antibiotics to fight infection. The prognosis is usually good if pressure within the skull can be controlled.

Ischemic optic neuropathy

Ischemic optic neuropathy is a painless swelling of the optic nerve due to reduced blood supply. This can lead to impaired neural function or the death of nerve cells. The amount of vision loss varies but may be severe and permanent. The loss can occur over minutes and hours, or it may develop gradually over several days. Both eyes can be involved.

The condition most often develops in adults age 50 and older. It may be associated with an underlying chronic condition, such as high blood pressure, atherosclerosis or diabetes. It may also result from inflammation of certain arteries in the head (temporal arteritis).

Treatment involves managing factors, such as blood pressure and cholesterol, that affect blood supply to the optic nerve. Corticosteroid medications may be administered if the condition is a result of temporal arteritis.

5

Glaucoma

Glaucoma is sometimes called the silent thief of sight. That's because the most common form of the disease develops with no warning signs. The damage is so gradual that many people don't realize they have any vision loss until the disease is in an advanced stage.

Glaucoma is also unrelenting and tenacious. The number of people who have this condition continues to increase worldwide and is currently estimated at 80 million. Glaucoma is the leading cause of irreversible blindness worldwide and the second most common cause of vision loss in the United States, after age-related macular degeneration.

Actually, glaucoma is not one disease but a group of related eye conditions. The feature they all have in common is damage to the optic nerve, the bundle of nerve fibers that carries signals between the eye and the brain. Abnormally high pressure inside your eye (intraocular pressure) is usually what damages the optic nerve.

As the optic nerve deteriorates, blind spots develop in your visual field, typically starting with your side (peripheral) vision. The exact cause of glaucoma isn't known, but several factors may be involved, including inflammation and vascular, mechanical and even neurological problems.

Fortunately, only a small number of people with glaucoma ever lose their sight completely. That's because medical advances have made the condition easier to detect and treat. If caught early, glaucoma may never cause detectable vision loss. But having glaucoma does require regular monitoring and treatment for the rest of your life.

CELL DAMAGE AND DEATH

Vision loss associated with glaucoma is the result of disrupted communication due to cell damage in the optic nerve. Because of the damage, electrical signals can't move freely between the retina and the brain's visual cortex. It's unclear why, but when optic nerve cells are damaged, they inevitably die rather than stabilize or repair themselves. Researchers are trying to understand how this process occurs.

What causes cell damage in the optic nerve is a topic of debate. One theory holds that abnormally high eye pressure causes structural damage in the optic nerve. Another theory proposes that increased eye pressure blocks small blood vessels feeding the optic nerve, starving the nerve cells. A more recent theory suggests an imbalance between eye pressure and brain pressure inhibits the flow of molecules from the brain necessary for eye health.

Having increased pressure within an eye puts you at a greatly increased risk of glaucoma. However, high intraocular pressure doesn't mean that you have glaucoma. Some people are better able to tolerate increased eye pressure than are others, without experiencing optic nerve damage. It's also possible to develop glaucoma even if your eye pressure is within the range of what's considered normal — between 10 and 21 millimeters of mercury (mm Hg). For this reason, eye pressure may only be one contributing factor in the disease process.

To better understand the connections between eye pressure and glaucoma, it's helpful to know more about the mechanisms that regulate intraocular pressure and what may cause the pressure to rise.

Changes in pressure are connected to the flow of aqueous humor circulating through the front part of your eye. Aqueous humor is a transparent fluid produced within the eye. It circulates through the eye's anterior chamber and around the lens and cornea before draining away (see the illustration on the opposite page). Continuous flow of aqueous humor nourishes the eye and removes unwanted debris.

Aqueous humor exits the eye through a drainage system located at the narrow angle where the iris and the cornea meet. Here, fluid passes through spongy tissue known as the trabecular meshwork. It then drains into an open channel called Schlemm's canal and is eventually absorbed into the body's bloodstream. Your eye produces aqueous humor at about the

Eye pressure

Internal eye pressure (intraocular pressure) allows the eye to hold its shape and to function properly. Think of intraocular pressure as air in a balloon — the right amount of pressure keeps the balloon round and taut, whereas too much pressure may subject it to damage.

same rate as the amount of fluid that drains out of the anterior chamber.

When the drainage system doesn't function properly — for example, the meshwork becomes clogged — exit of aqueous humor from the eye becomes more difficult. Drainage resistance is almost always the cause of elevated intraocular pressure. There are occasions

when the trabecular meshwork is blocked completely. Total blockage creates an emergency situation with a rapid, extreme increase in eye pressure.

TYPES

There are several types of glaucoma. The differences have to do with what's

INTRAOCULAR PRESSURE

The flow of aqueous humor through the anterior chamber at the front of the eye plays an important role in controlling your intraocular pressure. Aqueous humor exits the eye through the trabecular meshwork, located where the iris and cornea meet (see inset). The fluid filters through the meshwork before passing into an open channel called Schlemm's canal. Increased resistance to flow aqueous humor at the trabecular meshwork can increase eye pressure.

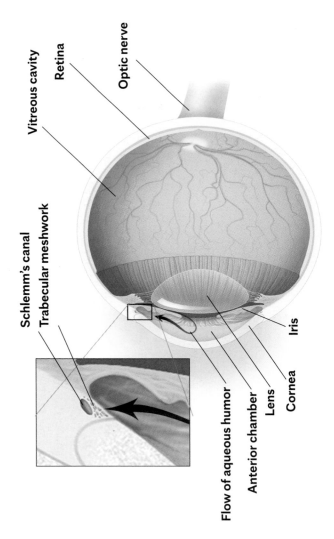

Schlemm's canal
Trabecular meshwork
Vitreous cavity
Retina
Optic nerve
Iris
Flow of aqueous humor
Anterior chamber
Lens
Cornea

inhibiting aqueous humor from draining out of the anterior chamber.

Open-angle

Open-angle glaucoma is the most common form of the disease. The drainage angle formed by the cornea and iris remains open, but the trabecular meshwork is partially blocked. This causes pressure in the eye to gradually increase. The increase in pressure damages the optic nerve.

Damage to the optic nerve is slow and painless. A large part of your vision can be lost before you're even aware that there's a problem.

What causes the blockage in open-angle glaucoma is unknown. It may be age-related — aqueous humor drains less efficiently as you get older. But that may be only part of the equation because not all older adults develop this form of glaucoma. The condition also may be genetic — it's more common in individuals who have a family history of glaucoma.

Angle-closure

Angle-closure glaucoma, also called closed-angle glaucoma, occurs when the iris bulges forward to narrow or block the drainage angle formed by the cornea and iris, making it more difficult for aqueous humor to drain away.

This angle is the pathway for aqueous humor to reach the trabecular meshwork.

In a chronic form of this disease, the iris forms scar tissue over the meshwork, permanently closing off parts of the drainage pathway. As fluid backs up, pressure within the eye increases.

Though not as prevalent as the open-angle form, angle-closure glaucoma is more common among farsighted individuals, who tend to have smaller eyes, and among certain racial or ethnic groups, including Asians. As you get older, your lens becomes larger, pushing the iris forward and narrowing the angle.

Sometimes, the pathway closes off completely and suddenly, blocking aqueous humor from reaching the trabecular meshwork at all, and causing a sudden increase in eye pressure. This is known as acute angle-closure glaucoma.

Acute angle-closure glaucoma can occur if the pupils become widened (dilated) in a person whose eyes already have a narrow drainage angle. Certain factors that may cause your pupils to dilate include:

• Darkness or dim light
• Stress or excitement
• Certain medications, such as antihistamines and tricyclic antidepressants
• Eye drops used to dilate the pupils, for example, during an eye exam — dilating eye drops may not cause the angle to close until several hours after they're put in.

Acute angle-closure glaucoma is a medical emergency requiring immediate treatment. The condition can cause vision loss within hours of its onset, and without treatment, blindness can develop in the eye in as little as one or two days. Although an acute attack often affects only one eye, the other eye becomes at higher risk of attack.

Normal-tension

In normal-tension glaucoma, also known as low-tension glaucoma, your optic nerve becomes damaged even though your eye pressure is within the normal range. Damage to the optic nerve occurs in a pattern consistent with glaucoma.

OPEN-ANGLE GLAUCOMA

Blockage of the trabecular meshwork slows the drainage of aqueous humor out of the eye. This causes a buildup of fluid in the anterior chamber and gradual increase of intraocular pressure.

Normal-tension glaucoma is a poorly understood, though not uncommon, form of the disease. Why damage occurs is unknown. It's possible you may have a sensitive or fragile optic nerve, in which even normal amounts of pressure can damage it.

Or your optic nerve may be receiving a reduced amount of blood. Limited blood flow may be associated with atherosclerosis — the buildup of fatty deposits (plaques) in the arteries — or other conditions that may impair circulation, such as abnormally low blood pressure.

ANGLE-CLOSURE GLAUCOMA

With the acute form, the angle formed by the cornea and the iris closes completely, blocking aqueous humor from draining out of the eye. This causes a sudden, rapid increase in intraocular pressure.

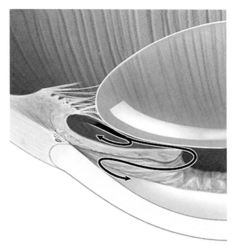

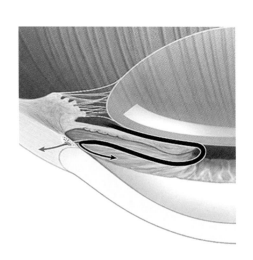

Secondary

Glaucoma is referred to as secondary when it's a complication of another medical condition. (Glaucoma is a primary condition when the cause is unknown.) Secondary glaucoma may stem from a variety of diseases, medications, physical injuries or trauma, and eye inflammation or abnormalities. Infrequently, eye surgery can cause secondary glaucoma.

Examples of secondary glaucoma include pseudoexfoliative glaucoma, which occurs when small particles produced in the eye accumulate and block the trabecular meshwork, and neovascular glaucoma, associated with diabetes.

SIGNS AND SYMPTOMS

The most common forms of glaucoma — open-angle glaucoma and chronic angle-closure glaucoma — typically occur with few if any symptoms until they reach a more advanced stage. Although at first you may notice vision problems in just one eye, eventually the condition affects both eyes.

As nerve damage progresses, you gradually lose your peripheral vision. You may have trouble seeing objects off to the side or out of the corner of your eye, and over time it may start to feel as if you're looking through a tunnel. Other symptoms include trouble differentiating

DAMAGE TO THE OPTIC DISK

Evidence of glaucoma includes damaged nerve fibers in the optic nerve, causing the optic disk to appear cupped or excavated.

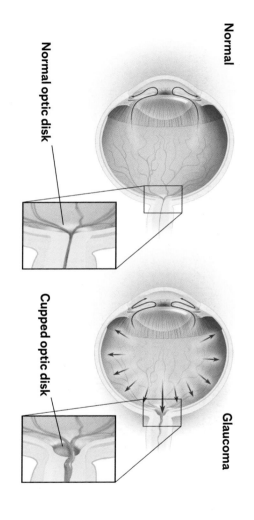

Normal

Normal optic disk

Glaucoma

Cupped optic disk

between varying shades of light and dark, and difficulty seeing at night.

Acute angle-closure glaucoma, you'll recall, results from a sudden and rapid increase in internal eye pressure. An attack often happens in situations when your pupils become dilated, such as at night in a room with dim lighting.

Emergency signs and symptoms include:
• Blurred vision
• Halos around lights
• Reddening of the eye
• Severe headache or eye pain
• Nausea and vomiting

If any of these signs or symptoms occur, seek immediate medical attention.

Permanent vision loss can happen within hours of the attack.

Signs and symptoms of secondary glaucoma will vary, depending on what's causing the glaucoma and whether the drainage angle remains open or closed.

RISK FACTORS

If your intraocular pressure is above what's considered normal — between 10 and 21 mm Hg — you're at higher risk of glaucoma. However, not everyone with elevated intraocular pressure develops the disease. This makes it difficult to predict who will or will not experience glaucoma.

VISION WITH GLAUCOMA

The gradual loss of peripheral vision is portrayed in this sequence from normal visual field (left) to early-stage glaucoma (center) to advanced-stage glaucoma (right). Your brain fills in the details so that missing areas of vision go unnoticed.

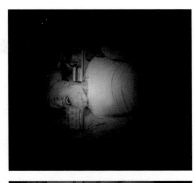
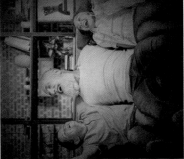
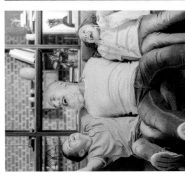

The following factors also are known to increase your risk of glaucoma. Because chronic forms can destroy vision before symptoms are apparent, it's important to be aware of all risk factors.

- **Age.** Open-angle glaucoma is rare before age 40, but everyone older than 60 is at increased risk of glaucoma.
- **Race and ethnicity.** Being Black, Asian or Hispanic increases your risk. The reasons why aren't clear.
- **Family history.** If a member in your immediate family (parent, sibling) has glaucoma, you're at greater risk of developing the disease. This suggests a defect in one or more genes may make certain individuals more susceptible.
- **Medical conditions.** Diabetes, high blood pressure, heart disease and hypothyroidism increase your risk of developing glaucoma. Other risk factors include vascular problems, such as stroke and Raynaud's disease, and inflammatory eye conditions, such as chronic uveitis and iritis.
- **Physical injuries.** Severe trauma, such as a blow to the eye, may result in elevated eye pressure. An injury can also dislocate the lens, closing the drainage angle.
- **Extreme nearsightedness and far-sightedness.** These conditions can increase your risk of glaucoma.
- **Prolonged corticosteroid use.** Corticosteroid eye drops, inhalers or pills may put certain individuals at risk of increased intraocular pressure.
- **Eye abnormalities.** Abnormalities in the structure of the eye may cause secondary glaucoma. Previous eye surgery also may trigger secondary glaucoma.

SCREENING

Routine eye exams are key to detecting glaucoma at an early stage and experiencing successful treatment. If you have one or more risk factors for glaucoma, talk to your eye doctor regarding regular eye appointments.

As a general rule, the American Academy of Ophthalmology recommends having a comprehensive eye exam:

- Every 5 to 10 years if you're under 40 years old
- Every 2 to 4 years if you're 40 to 54 years old
- Every 1 to 3 years if you're 55 to 64 years old
- Every 1 to 2 years if you're older than age 65

If you're at risk of glaucoma, you'll need more-frequent screenings. If you're being treated for glaucoma, establish a regular schedule of eye examinations to make sure your intraocular eye pressure remains at safe levels.

Be alert for the symptoms of acute angle-closure glaucoma, such as severe headache or severe pain in your eye or eyebrow, nausea, blurred vision, or seeing rainbow halos around lights. If you experience any of these symptoms, seek immediate medical care.

DIAGNOSING GLAUCOMA

No single test can determine conclusively that you have glaucoma. A diagnosis is based on indications of damage to the optic nerve. If you have glaucoma, when an eye doctor examines your retina the optic disk will appear indented (excavated), as if someone has scooped out part of its center. This is known as cupping and it results from the death of nerve cells. Loss of nerve cells may also affect the normal contour and color of the optic disk.

Other factors that may indicate the development of glaucoma include elevated intraocular pressure and areas of vision loss. Abnormally high intraocular pressure is frequently, but not always, associated with glaucoma. Generally, the disease is accompanied by a gradual loss of peripheral vision.

Several tests, some of which are commonly performed during regular eye exams, are used in the diagnosis of glaucoma.

Tonometry

Tonometry is a simple, painless procedure that measures your intraocular pressure. It's typically the initial screening test for glaucoma (see page 27).

For the test, an eye specialist will ask you to sit before a slit lamp, where a small flat-tipped cone pushes lightly against the cornea of your eyeball. The force required to flatten (applanate) a small area of your cornea translates into a measure of your intraocular pressure.

A variety of factors may cause slight variation in tonometry readings from one person to the next. These factors include the thickness of your cornea and whether you've had corneal laser surgery, such as LASIK. To account for the variation, newer technologies are being investigated that may improve the standard applanation instrument and obtain more-accurate intraocular pressure measurements.

Visual field test (perimetry)

This exam can determine if glaucoma has affected your visual field (see page 22). For the test, you're seated in front of a lighted bowl on which bright points of light flash on and off. You'll be asked to press a button whenever you notice one of these flashes. Your responses are analyzed and used to map your entire visual field.

Optic nerve exam

An instrument called an ophthalmoscope, or biomicroscope, is used to determine the health of your optic nerve. This instrument allows your eye doctor to look directly through your pupil to the back of your eye. He or she is looking for evidence of cupping on the optic disk.

Your eye doctor may also use imaging techniques such as optical coherence tomography (OCT) to create a 3D image of your optic nerve (see page 52). This test can reveal very slight changes to the nerve fibers, providing early evidence that glaucoma may be developing.

Before the exam is complete, a photograph may be taken of the optic disk. The image can be used for comparison at future visits and help monitor changes to the optic disk.

Pachymetry

To accurately diagnose glaucoma, the thickness of your cornea — the transparent, protective dome located at the front of your eye — also is considered. Generally, thin corneas produce artificially low intraocular pressure readings, masking glaucoma risk. Conversely, thick corneas produce artificially high intraocular pressure readings, causing unnecessary concern.

Your doctor may perform a test called pachymetry that uses ultrasound to gauge the cornea's thickness. With this measurement, your intraocular pressure can be calculated correctly.

Gonioscopy

This test is performed to evaluate the internal drainage system of the eye, also known as the anterior chamber angle. It involves a special lens to inspect the drainage angle where your iris and cornea meet. A blocked angle could mean angle-closure glaucoma. No blockage may indicate open-angle glaucoma.

VISUAL FIELD MAP

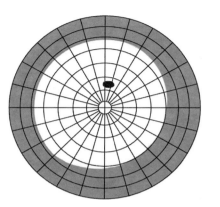

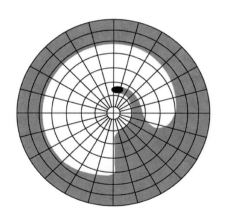

A normal visual field of the left eye mapped by tangent screen perimetry (see page 22) is shown at left. The black spot near the center marks your normal blind spot — the location of the optic nerve. The visual field at right (also a left eye) shows a typical pattern associated with glaucoma. Shading indicates that the upper right portion of the visual field has been lost.

COMBINING TESTS RESULTS

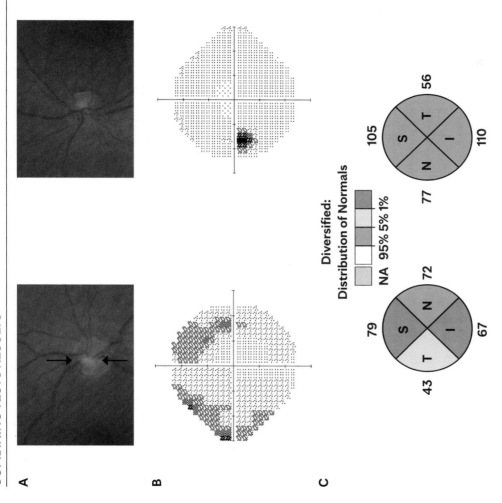

Diversified:
Distribution of Normals

NA   95%   5%   1%

These images show how several test results may be used to make a diagnosis. All come from the same person. In the top row (A), note the larger optic nerve cup in the left image (see arrows). The second row (B) shows results of a visual field test (automated perimetry). Gray areas in the left image indicate visual field loss consistent with glaucoma. The bottom row (C) shows the results of a test called optical coherence tomography (OCT). The red and yellow shading in the left image indicates thinning of the retinal nerve fiber layer consistent with glaucoma, compared with no thinning in the right image.

There is no cure for glaucoma, and damage to your vision caused by the disease can't be reversed. The good news is, with treatment, glaucoma can usually be managed, reducing the risk of further progression of the disease.

The best way to preserve your existing vision is by controlling your intraocular pressure — either by improving the drainage of aqueous humor from your eye or by reducing its production within your eye, or both.

The results of your eye exam will help guide the course of treatment:

• If you have a cupped optic disk, that most likely means you'll be treated for glaucoma.

• If you have signs of optic nerve damage and visual field loss, even if your intraocular pressure is within a normal range, you may receive treatment to reduce your eye pressure and try to slow progression of the disease.

• If you have only slightly elevated intraocular pressure, an undamaged optic nerve and no loss of visual field, treatment may not be necessary, but you'll need frequent eye exams to monitor your condition.

When deciding on your treatment, your doctor may take other factors into consideration, such as your overall physical health, psychosocial issues and risk of side effects. Because glaucoma can subtly change, treatment may need to be adjusted. Regular checkups and adherence to your treatment plan may seem burdensome, but they're essential to preventing vision loss.

To treat glaucoma, your doctor may prescribe eye drops, oral medications, laser treatment, surgery or a combination of these therapies. Topical medications applied directly to the eye are the most common initial treatment. Surgery may be recommended if medications are ineffective or if the person taking them has difficulty complying with the recommended therapy. Surgery also can be a relatively safe and effective initial treatment.

Eye drops

Medicated eye drops are often the first step in treating glaucoma. There are a variety of eye drops that your eye doctor may prescribe (see pages 102-103). When a single medication isn't effective, a combination medication or multiple medications may be prescribed.

It's important to use the eye drops exactly as prescribed. Skipping even a few doses may worsen optic nerve damage. Some eye drops need to be applied several times each day, while others are used just once daily. Make sure to let your doctor know of other medications you take to avoid any drug interactions.

Because some eye drop fluid is absorbed into your bloodstream, you may experience side effects unrelated to your eyes. To minimize this absorption, close your eyes for a minute or two after putting the drops in. Press lightly at the corner of your eye near your nose to close the tear duct, and then wipe off unused fluid from your eyelid.

Oral medications

If eye drops alone don't reduce your eye pressure to your target level, your doctor may prescribe an oral medication. Oral medications are generally considered a short-term option as part of an overall treatment plan.

The most common oral medications for glaucoma are carbonic anhydrase inhibitors. They include acetazolamide and methazolamide. These medications are taken with meals to reduce their side effects. To minimize potassium loss often associated with the medications, add bananas and apple juice to your diet.

When you start taking these medications, you may experience a frequent need to urinate and a tingling sensation in your fingers and toes. These symptoms will usually disappear after a few days. Other possible side effects include rashes, depression, fatigue, lethargy, kidney stones, stomach upset, impotence, weight loss and a metallic taste in your mouth when drinking carbonated beverages.

Neuroprotective drugs

Reducing your eye's intraocular pressure to a target level is generally considered effective at minimizing vision loss from glaucoma. But, sometimes, vision loss occurs even when the intraocular pressure is within a normal range, indicating that factors other than pressure are involved.

DETERMINING YOUR TARGET PRESSURE

As part of your treatment plan, your eye doctor will identify your baseline intraocular pressure. This may be achieved by measuring your intraocular pressure several times and at different times of the day.

Once your baseline pressure has been determined, the next step is to identify your target pressure — a lower intraocular pressure level that's unlikely to cause further damage to the optic nerve. Your target pressure may be a range rather than a single number. This is the pressure level that you want to achieve with treatment.

Your doctor will consider whether you have optic nerve damage and other factors in determining your target pressure. In addition, your target pressure may change over the course of your lifetime.

EYE DROPS FOR GLAUCOMA

Your eye doctor may prescribe more than one type of eye drop. If you're using different types, wait several minutes between applications of each type. The types of eye drops that doctors most commonly prescribe include:

Type	Function	Drug names
Beta blockers	Reduce the production of fluid (aqueous humor) in the eye and lower intraocular pressure	Betaxolol (Betoptic S), carteolol, levobunolol (Akbeta, Betagan), timolol (Betimol, Istalol, Timoptic)
Alpha-adrenergic agents	Reduce the production of aqueous humor and increase drainage of fluid from the eye	Apraclonidine (Iopidine), brimonidine (Alphagan P, Qoliana)
Carbonic anhydrase inhibitors	Reduce the production of aqueous humor	Brinzolamide (Azopt), dorzolamide (Trusopt)
Prostaglandins	Increase the drainage of fluid from the eye	Bimatoprost (Lumigan), latanoprost (Xalatan), tafluprost (Zioptan), travoprost (Travatan Z), latanoprostene bunod (Vyzulta)
Rho kinase inhibitors	Increase the drainage of fluid from the eye	Netarsudil (Rhopressa)
Miotics (uncommonly used today)	Increase the drainage of fluid from the eye	Pilocarpine (Isopto Carpine)
Combination eye drops	Usually prescribed instead of separate medications if more than one type is necessary to control intraocular pressure	Timolol/dorzolamide (Cosopt); timolol/brimonidine (Combigan); brimonidine/brinzolamide (Simbrinza); netarsudil/latanoprost (Rocklatan)

Possible side effects

Possible side effects
Burning and stinging upon use; blurred vision, dry eye, tearing, itching and the sensation of a foreign body in the eye, as well as dizziness; different medications may be recommended if you have asthma, chronic obstructive pulmonary disease, heart failure or diabetes
Itching, tearing, eye discomfort, swelling of the eyelid, dry mouth and the sensation of a foreign body in the eye; also irregular heart rate, high blood pressure, fatigue and dizziness
Blurred vision, changes in taste, burning and stinging, and dryness; when medication is taken orally, frequent urination and a tingling sensation in the fingers and toes are common; if you're allergic or sensitive to sulfa drugs, this medication shouldn't be used unless there's no alternative, and then only with care
Blurred vision, burning and stinging, itching, pain, the sensation of a foreign body in the eye, increased pigmentation of the iris, and longer, thicker eyelashes
Redness, bursting of the small blood vessels on the surface of the eye that may cause redness and blurred vision
Burning and discomfort upon use; tearing, blurred vision, headache, and nearsightedness (all more common for initial use); increased salivation and digestive problems may rarely occur
Identical side effects to those of individual medications (see listings above); Simbrinza may be a good choice for people with medical concerns associated with beta blockers

Researchers are exploring neuroprotective approaches to treating the optic nerve. Clinical trials have examined whether drugs such as memantine (Namenda) may protect nerve fibers from damage. So far, they've been inconclusive.

Laser therapy

A procedure called trabeculoplasty may be used to treat open-angle glaucoma when medications aren't effective or are causing troublesome side effects. For the procedure, a high-energy laser beam stimulates the trabecular meshwork, reducing fluid resistance and lowering pressure. The laser energy is absorbed only by certain tissues, minimizing scarring.

Trabeculoplasty is an office procedure requiring 10 to 20 minutes to complete.

Most people can immediately resume normal activities without discomfort. However, it may take several weeks before a reduction in eye pressure is evident.

Laser therapy is as effective as the best glaucoma medications. The reduction in intraocular pressure laser therapy produces should remain for several years before gradually wearing off. The procedure may be repeated or different medications or surgery may be recommended.

Surgery

Surgery may be necessary to treat glaucoma if laser therapy or medications aren't effective or well tolerated. Surgery helps reduce resistance to the drainage of aqueous humor. However, it may not eliminate the need for medications.

EMERGENCY CARE FOR GLAUCOMA

Acute angle-closure glaucoma is a medical emergency. When you arrive at a hospital or clinic with this condition, doctors will attempt to reduce your eye pressure as quickly as possible using medications.

Once your eye pressure is under control, you may undergo a procedure called iridotomy. In this procedure, a surgeon uses a laser to create a small hole in your iris. This allows aqueous humor to flow more freely into the anterior chamber and have normal access to the trabecular meshwork.

If aqueous humor can once again reach the meshwork, normal drainage may be reestablished. Many doctors recommend an iridotomy on the other eye at a later date because of the high risk that it, too, will undergo an attack within the next few years.

Trabeculectomy

This procedure may be performed at a hospital or outpatient surgery center. A surgeon creates a small opening in the white of your eye (sclera) that allows excess fluid to drain into its outer layers. A small bubble (bleb) forms in the space between the sclera and the conjunctiva where excess aqueous humor collects. This fluid spreads out and is gradually absorbed by tiny capillaries in your eye. Fluid drainage helps reduce intraocular pressure.

Your doctor will monitor your eye pressure and eye health during several follow-up visits. He or she may prescribe antibiotic and anti-inflammatory eye drops to help fight infection and prevent scarring at the newly created opening.

Scarring can sometimes be a problem for younger individuals and among people who've previously undergone eye surgery. If needed, the sutures may be cut and anti-scarring medications may be injected to help improve intraocular pressure.

GLAUCOMA SURGERY

Trabeculectomy (left) creates an opening in the sclera to improve fluid drainage. A form of minimally invasive surgery (right) applies heat to open the trabecular meshwork.

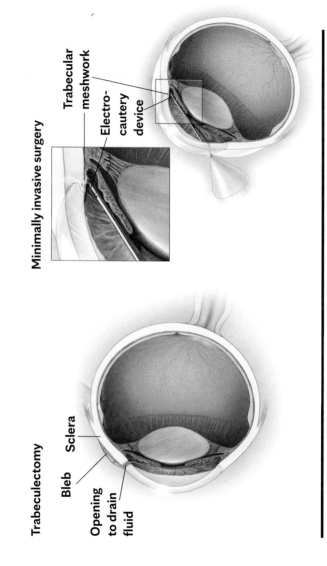

Trabeculectomy

Bleb Sclera

Opening to drain fluid

Minimally invasive surgery

Trabecular meshwork

Electro-cautery device

Another way to lower intraocular pressure is with drainage tubes. This approach may be taken if surgery has failed or if there's scarring or inflammation in the eye that makes other procedures unsuitable.

For the procedure, a surgeon inserts a small silicone tube into the anterior chamber at the front of your eye, which leads to a plastic plate on the sclera. The tube allows aqueous humor to drain from the chamber and be absorbed by tiny capillaries in the conjunctiva.

After surgery you'll wear an eye patch for 24 hours and need to use eye drops to fight infection and scarring. Plan on follow-up visits with your doctor afterward.

Minimally invasive surgery

New forms of surgery for treating glaucoma are available. These surgeries are characterized by smaller incisions, faster recovery and reduced risk of complications compared with traditional surgery. The disadvantage of minimally invasive procedures is that the reduction in intraocular pressure may not be as great as with trabeculectomy or a drainage tube.

Types of minimally invasive glaucoma surgery include trabecular meshwork removal, trabecular meshwork bypass, drainage to a bleb under the surface of the conjunctiva, or drainage to a space inside the eye called the suprachoroidal space. Some of these procedures may be combined with cataract surgery.

PREVENTION

Currently, there's no clear evidence that glaucoma can be prevented. However, some studies indicate possible benefits from use of certain medications and consuming certain foods. Further research is needed to confirm their value.

Other studies indicate that long-term use of cholesterol-lowering medications, such as statins, may reduce the risk of open-angle glaucoma, especially among people with cardiovascular disease. This may benefit individuals already taking the medications, but more study is necessary.

Regular comprehensive eye exams may be your best means of detecting glaucoma in its early stages. Follow the recommendations for eye checkups. To prevent the disease from progressing, it's important to keep yourself in good health and take your medications as prescribed.

General self-care tips to help prevent glaucoma include the following:

Eat a healthy diet

Consume plenty of fruits and vegetables to ensure that you're getting enough vitamins and minerals. Several nutrients are important to eye health, including zinc, copper, selenium, and antioxidant vitamins C, E and A.

Pay attention to fluids

Drink fluids regularly in small amounts over the course of a day. Drinking a quart or more of liquid within a short period of time may increase eye pressure. Limit caffeine to low or moderate levels. Drinking beverages with large amounts of caffeine may increase eye pressure.

Exercise carefully

People with open-angle glaucoma who exercise regularly may be able to moderately reduce intraocular pressure or risk of optic nerve damage. However, angle-closure glaucoma isn't affected by exercise.

A form of glaucoma known as pigmentary glaucoma may cause an increase in eye pressure after a workout. Certain forms of exercise, such as yoga, in which you're in a head-down position, aren't recommended because they can increase eye pressure. Discuss an appropriate exercise program with your doctor.

Sleep with your head elevated

Using a wedge pillow that keeps your head slightly raised, about 20 degrees, may help reduce intraocular pressure while you sleep.

Don't depend on herbal supplements

A number of herbal supplements are advertised as glaucoma remedies. They

shouldn't be used in place of other proven therapies. Be cautious and discuss herbal supplements with your doctor before trying them.

Manage stress

Excess or chronic stress can trigger an attack of acute angle-closure glaucoma. Relaxation techniques, such as meditation and progressive muscle relaxation, may help you manage stress.

Wear proper eye protection

Eye trauma can increase intraocular pressure. Wear safety glasses or goggles when playing sports, using tools or machinery, or working with chemicals. When out in the sun, even for a few minutes, wear sunglasses that block ultraviolet light.

6

Cataracts

A cataract is a clouding of the normally clear lens of your eye. The Latin word *cataract* means "waterfall" — alluding perhaps to the difficulty you might have trying to see through a sheet of white falling water. A better analogy might be trying to peer through a frosted or foggy window.

When a cataract clouds your vision, it becomes progressively more difficult to read, drive a car, enjoy a panoramic landscape, operate tools and appliances, use electronic devices, or recognize facial expressions.

As much as you may not wish to hear this news, understand that it's normal for the lens of your eye to cloud as you get older. It's likely that each one of us is on the way to developing a cataract. Most cataracts

develop slowly and generally don't disturb your eyesight early on. By age 80, however, more than half of all Americans either have cataracts or have had surgery to get rid of them.

How you deal with a cataract will depend on how severe the condition is and how well you tolerate blurred vision. In their early stages, cataracts are often left untreated because stronger lighting and eyeglasses help compensate for vision loss.

But at some point — when your vision becomes moderately to significantly impaired and jeopardizes your quality of life — you may need to seek treatment, which involves surgery. Fortunately, cataract removal is a safe, effective and common surgical procedure, restoring sight to millions of Americans.

TYPES

A cataract forms in the lens, a transparent structure located at the front of your eye. It can develop in one eye or in both eyes. And it may only affect part of the lens or the entire lens.

The lens is positioned just behind the colored iris, which can adjust to regulate how much light enters the eye. The lens is shaped much like a magnifying glass — thicker in the middle and thinner near the edges — and is suspended by a ring of fibrous ligaments.

When your eyes work properly, light passing through the cornea and pupil reaches the lens. The lens focuses the light, allowing it to converge at a central point. The focused light produces clear, sharp images on the retina, located on the back inside wall of your eyeball. The retina functions like the film of a camera.

When a cataract develops, the lens becomes clouded, scattering the light and preventing sharply defined images from focusing on the retina. The result is your vision becomes blurred. The greater the clouding, the greater the loss of vision.

There are three distinct layers of a lens (see illustration on page 112). And there are corresponding types of cataracts, identified by the layer of the lens where the clouding develops.

The outer layer of a lens is a thin membrane called the capsule. It surrounds a soft, clear material called the cortex. The hard center of the lens is the nucleus. If you think of the lens as a piece of fruit, the capsule is the skin, the cortex is the fleshy fruit, and the nucleus is the pit.

Each type of cataract may develop by itself, or it can form in combination with other types. And more than one type of

CATARACT MYTHS

Perhaps because cataracts are such a common eye disorder, there are many misconceptions about them. Here are some corrections:

- A cataract is not a film covering the outside of your eye. It develops within the eye, clouding the normally clear lens.
- Just because your eye looks clear doesn't mean there's no cataract. Most cataracts are detectable only with special instruments.
- Cataracts aren't caused by cancer.
- Cataracts don't spread from one eye to the other, although both eyes may be affected by cataracts.
- Overusing your eyes doesn't cause cataracts.
- You don't have to wait for a cataract to turn completely white or become "overripe" before having it removed.

cataract can develop in the lens at the same time.

Nuclear

A nuclear cataract develops in the center of the lens. It's the most common type of cataract and the one most associated with aging. Typical changes due to aging make the nucleus of the lens more compressed and less flexible.

Early on, as the lens changes the way it focuses light, you may experience an improvement in your reading vision. Some people actually stop needing their glasses. Unfortunately, this so-called second sight disappears as the lens gradually becomes discolored and clouds vision. As the cataract progresses, the lens may even turn brown. Seeing in dim light and driving at night can be difficult.

Cortical

A cortical cataract begins as whitish, wedge-shaped streaks that develop on the outer edge of the cortex layer. As the cataract progresses, the streaks extend to the center of the lens. Eventually, the clouding begins to interfere with light passing through the nucleus, impairing both distance and close-up vision. Difficulty focusing, distortion, problems with glare and loss of contrast may occur.

People with diabetes are at higher risk of developing cortical cataracts. Cortical

HOW A CATARACT AFFECT VISION

A cataract occurs when the normally clear lens of your eye becomes cloudy. The clouding blurs vision by scattering the light passing through the lens so that it can't properly focus an image on the retina.

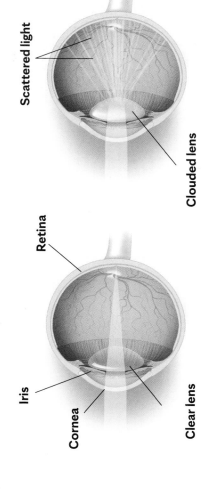

Iris

Retina

Scattered light

Cornea

Clouded lens

Clear lens

cataracts are the only type of cataract associated with exposure to ultraviolet (UV) light.

Subcapsular

A subcapsular cataract typically starts as a small, opaque area just under the capsule shell. It usually forms at the back of the lens, in the direct path of light on its way to the retina. A subcapsular cataract may occur in both eyes but tends to be more advanced in one eye than the other. This type of cataract may interfere with reading, reduce vision in bright light, and produce glare or halos around lights at night.

You're more likely to develop a subcapsular cataract if you have diabetes, are very

LAYERS OF THE LENS

A cataract may form in any one of the layers of the lens — the nucleus, the cortex or the capsule.

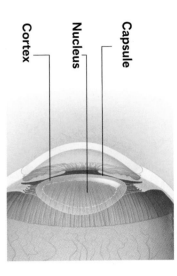

Capsule

Nucleus

Cortex

nearsighted, have taken corticosteroid drugs, or have had an eye injury, inflammation or surgery.

SIGNS AND SYMPTOMS

A cataract usually develops slowly and painlessly. At first, the cloudiness will affect only a small portion of the lens and you may be unaware of any vision changes. Over time, however, as the cataract grows and becomes larger, it affects more of the lens. When significantly less light is able to reach the retina due to the clouding, your vision becomes impaired.

Signs and symptoms of a cataract may include the following:

- Clouded, blurred or dim vision
- Difficulty with night vision
- Sensitivity to light and glare, which may become severe
- Seeing halos around lights
- Need for brighter light for reading and other activities
- Frequent changes in eyeglass or contact lens prescriptions
- Fading or yellowing of colors
- Double vision in one eye

Because of a cataract, sunlight, light from reading lamps or oncoming car headlights may appear too bright and intense. Glare and halos around lights can make driving at night uncomfortable and dangerous. You may experience eyestrain or eye fatigue or find yourself blinking more frequently to clear your vision.

Signs and symptoms such as pain, redness, itching, irritation or discharge aren't associated with a cataract but may be related to other eye disorders.

CAUSES

A cataract isn't dangerous to eye health unless it turns completely white (see page 114). This is known as an overripe (hyper-mature) cataract. A hypermature cataract may rupture, causing inflammation, pain, headache and possibly glaucoma. Hyper-mature cataracts are rare and should be removed as quickly as possible.

The eye's lens is made mostly of water and protein fibers. The protein fibers are precisely arranged to allow light to pass through the lens without interference. As you age, the composition of the lens changes and the structure of the protein fibers breaks down. Some of the fibers clump together, clouding small areas of the lens. The lens also becomes thicker

VISION WITH A CATARACT

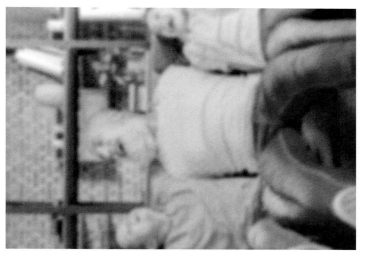
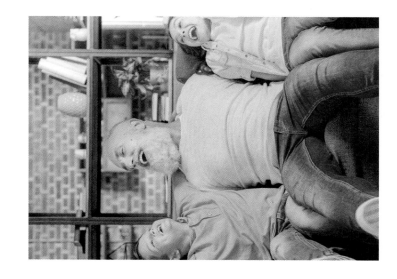

A clouded lens from a cataract progressively turns clear vision (left) into blurred or dimmed vision (right).

and less flexible. As a cataract develops, the clouding becomes denser, involving a larger area of the lens.

Scientists don't know why these changes occur. One possibility could be damage from unstable molecules known as free radicals. Smoking and exposure to ultraviolet light are two sources of free radicals. General wear and tear on the lens also may produce changes.

You don't have to be an older adult to develop cataracts — they can start at an early age. But such cataracts tend to be small and develop slowly, often not affecting vision until age 60 or older.

HYPERMATURE CATARACT

An overripe (hypermature) cataract occurs when a lens becomes completely clouded, giving the pupil a white appearance. The condition is rare and should be treated immediately.

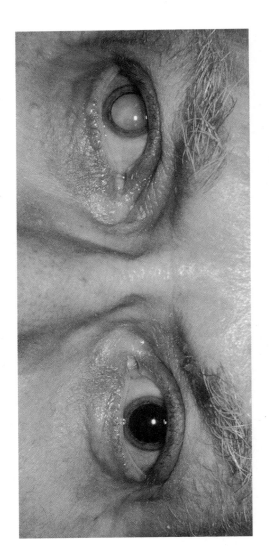

Some children are born with cataracts, while others develop cataracts during childhood. Most of these cataracts don't affect vision, but some may interfere with the neural connections that form between a child's eyes and brain in the first years of life, which can cause permanent vision loss. See Chapter 8 for more information.

RISK FACTORS

Everyone is at risk of developing cataracts simply because age is such a prominent factor. By age 75 most individuals have developed some degree of lens clouding, although it may not impair vision. Cataracts are slightly more common in women than in men, and they're more common in white people than in Black people or people who are Hispanic.

Other factors that may increase your risk of cataracts include:

- Diabetes
- Family history of cataracts
- Previous eye surgery
- Previous eye injury or inflammation
- Prolonged use of corticosteroids
- Excessive exposure to sunlight
- Smoking
- Excessive consumption of alcohol

SCREENING AND DIAGNOSIS

A complete eye exam is the only way to know if you have a cataract. During the exam, your pupils are dilated with special drops, which allows your eye doctor to look for signs of a cataract on the lens. If signs are visible, your doctor can determine how dense the clouding is.

If a cataract is impairing your vision, you can discuss treatment options with your doctor. If, in addition to a cataract, you have another serious eye condition, you'll need to be prepared for the possibility that removing the cataract may not improve your vision.

SURGERY

The only effective treatment for a well-established cataract is surgery. During the procedure, a surgeon removes the

clouded lens and replaces it with an artificial lens implant that restores clear vision. Cataracts can't be cured with medications, dietary supplements, exercise or optical devices.

In the early stages of a cataract, treatment involves helping you find ways to cope with your symptoms. Having a good understanding of the condition and a willingness to adapt are vital.

Here are steps for dealing with symptoms:

- If you have eyeglasses or contact lenses, make sure they're the most accurate prescription possible.
- Use a magnifying glass to read.
- Improve the lighting in your home with more or brighter lamps, for example, ones that can accommodate halogen lights or 100- to 150-watt incandescent bulbs.
- When you're outside during the day, wear sunglasses to reduce glare.
- Limit your night driving.

These measures are likely to help you compensate for vision loss for a while, but as the cataract progresses, your sight will continue to deteriorate.

Doctors recommend surgery when the reduction in your vision starts to interfere with your ability to perform daily activities and it affects your quality of life. Here are some questions to consider: Does your cataract prevent you from reading, watching TV or driving a car? Is it difficult to use kitchen utensils and appliances? Can you move around the house safely or go up and down steps without fear of falling?

If you answered yes to any of these questions, it may be time to consider surgery. Most people who undergo cataract surgery enjoy improved vision and quality of life. Cataract surgery is one of the most common operations performed in the United States.

Determining the right time for surgery

The decision to have cataract surgery is one that you and your eye doctor will make together. Generally, there is no rush, so take time to consider your options carefully.

AN EYE ON HISTORY

Decades ago, cataract surgery was a major ordeal that included several days in the hospital, painful stitches in the eye, and a recovery process that included lying on your back with your head held in place with sandbags. In addition, thick glasses replaced the focusing power of the internal lens. Luckily, the procedure has changed dramatically for the better.

Modern day surgical treatment started with the development of the intraocular lens in 1949 by Nicholas Harold Ridley, M.D., an English ophthalmologist. Dr. Ridley recalled the experiences of eye doctors who had treated Royal Air Force pilots during World War II. Some pilots had tiny shards of hard plastic lodged in their eyes after their planes' cockpits shattered. To the doctors' surprise, these fragments didn't cause serious problems in the pilots' eyes, even if they remained in place for long periods of time. With this in mind, Dr. Ridley began experimenting with making artificial lenses from plastic that could be implanted in the eye.

In the mid-1960s, American ophthalmologist Charles Kelman, M.D., developed phacoemulsification, a surgical procedure in which ultrasound technology removes the cataract while leaving the capsule surrounding the lens in place. This could be achieved with a small incision and minor intrusion into the delicate structure of the lens, greatly reducing recovery time.

Advances in surgical techniques and artificial lens design have made cataract surgery one of the safest and most effective surgical procedures. Millions of cataract surgeries are performed each year, and that number is expected to increase as the general population ages.

What might the future hold? One area of development is the creation of intraocular lenses with the ability to accommodate visual changes.

In most cases, waiting until you feel ready to have surgery won't damage your eye. The rate at which a cataract typically develops means you may not need surgery for many years, if at all. Among people with diabetes, however, cataracts may develop more quickly.

Base your decision on your degree of vision loss and your ability to function. How active are you, and does lack of vision affect your independence?

PHACOEMULSIFICATION

During the phacoemulsification procedure, the rapidly vibrating tip of an ultrasound probe breaks up the cataract, which a surgeon then suctions out (top). After removing the clouded lens, the surgeon delicately inserts a lens implant into the empty capsule that remains following the procedure (bottom).

Answers to these questions vary. A retired adult may have less need for sharp vision than a younger, more active adult. The retiree may choose to delay treatment, whereas the younger individual with less vision loss may elect to have surgery because of problems such as glare or double vision.

Sometimes, surgery may be necessary even if it's not causing serious vision loss. For example, a cataract may be removed if it's interfering with treatment of age-related macular degeneration, diabetic retinopathy or retinal detachment.

If you have cataracts in both eyes, the cataracts are removed one at a time in separate surgeries. This allows the first eye to heal properly before the second surgery takes place. More people are choosing to have cataract surgery on the second eye much sooner and more frequently than in the past, often within a few months of the first procedure.

The surgical procedure

Careful preparation is necessary prior to surgery to determine the correct focal power of your lens implant. Your surgeon will measure the size of your eyeball (axial length), along with the refractive properties of your cornea and the intended position of the artificial lens implant. Precise measurements are typically made using sophisticated technology known as laser interferometry.

Cataract surgery is typically an outpatient procedure that takes less than an

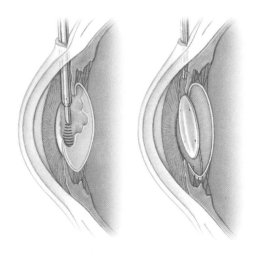

hour. Most people need only local anesthesia and are relaxed and comfortable during the surgery. On rare occasions, some people may need to be put under general anesthesia.

Different approaches may be used to remove a cataract.

Phacoemulsification

The most commonly used form of cataract surgery is called phacoemulsification (see page 117). During this procedure, the cataract is broken up and removed while leaving most of the outer layer of the lens (capsule) in place. The capsule provides support for the lens implant after the implant is inserted in the eye.

A small incision is made in the outer layer of the eyeball. A needle-thin ultrasound probe is inserted through the incision. Working inside the lens, a surgeon uses ultrasound waves to break up (emulsify) the cataract. The fragments are then suctioned out.

INTRAOCULAR LENS OPTIONS

A variety of lens implants (intraocular lenses) are available to replace natural lenses that have been blurred by cataracts. Prior to surgery, discuss your options carefully with your ophthalmologist. Depending on your needs, some options may be better for you than others.

Implantable lenses can be divided into three basic categories:

Monofocal lenses. They have a fixed point of focus for either near vision or distance vision. If a distance lens is implanted, you'll need to wear glasses or contact lenses for reading; if a near-vision lens is implanted, you'll need glasses for driving. Most monofocal lenses implanted for cataracts correct for distance vision and are supplemented by reading glasses.

Multifocal lenses. These lenses are much like bifocal or progressive lenses used in eyeglasses. With multifocal lenses, you may not need to wear corrective lenses after surgery, at least for most tasks. These intraocular lenses are designed to allow you to see well at distances both near and far. However, some people with multifocal lenses experience problems with glare, halos around lights and reduced sharpness of vision (contrast sensitivity), especially at night or in dim light. In addition, your distance vision with a multifocal intraocular lens may improve but perhaps not as much as with a monofocal intraocular lens that corrects for distance.

Extracapsular cataract extraction

Another surgical procedure is extracapsular cataract extraction. Using a larger incision than is made for phacoemulsification, a surgeon opens the lens capsule, removes the nucleus in one piece and vacuums out the lens cortex, leaving the capsule shell in place. Due to a greater risk of complications, this procedure is performed only in special circumstances.

With both procedures, once the cataract has been removed, an artificial lens is implanted into the empty lens capsule to replace the clouded lens. This lens implant, known as an intraocular lens, is made of plastic, acrylic or silicone and becomes a permanent part of your eye.

There are different types of intraocular lenses. Some are rigid and implanted through incisions that require stitches to close. Many intraocular lenses are flexible, allowing placement through smaller incisions. The surgeon folds the lenses and inserts them into the capsules where they unfold in place.

Toric intraocular lenses. These lenses attempt to minimize dependence on eyeglasses to correct astigmatism. Among people who have astigmatism, the clear front part of the eye (cornea) is shaped like a football instead of a basketball. A toric intraocular lens implant is football shaped. It helps counteract or negate corneal astigmatism and minimize the need for eyeglasses to correct astigmatism after cataract surgery.

Other options you and your eye doctor may consider include:

Limbal relaxing incisions. Another way for your surgeon to treat astigmatism during cataract surgery is to create small incisions at the edges of the cornea that allow its shape to be rounder and more symmetrical. This may be a good option if you have a high degree of astigmatism and prefer multifocal intraocular lenses.

Monovision. To avoid the need for reading glasses, your eye doctor may suggest monofocal lenses with a twist. One eye (usually your dominant eye) is corrected for distance, and the other eye is corrected for near vision. This is referred to as monovision. Its success depends on your brain's ability to pay attention only to the eye with the clear focus and ignore the blurry image from the other eye. If you've had monovision contact lenses before, this may be a good option for you.

After cataract surgery

With phacoemulsification and foldable implants, surgical incisions are typically small and often require no stitches. If all goes well, you'll heal quickly. If surgery requires a larger incision and stitches, healing may take a little longer.

Typically, you can go home on the day of your surgery, but you won't be able to drive, so arrange for a ride home beforehand. Your eye doctor may schedule a follow-up visit within a day of surgery. To monitor whether the surgical site is healing and your sight is improving, your doctor may also want to check on you once or twice more over the next month.

Healing generally takes 4 to 6 weeks. During this time, it's typical to experience mild eye discomfort. Avoid rubbing or pressing on your eye. Clean your eyelid with soft tissue or cotton balls to remove any crusty discharge.

As your eye heals, you may experience the following signs and symptoms:

- Blurry vision
- Secretions from the eye
- Itching
- Mild tearing

SECONDARY CATARACTS

During routine cataract surgery, the back (posterior) half of the lens capsule typically remains, and this structure is used to support the lens implant after the implant is put in place. A secondary cataract, or "after cataract," may develop when the capsule membrane turns cloudy, obscuring vision to a similar degree as the original cataract. Another term for this condition is posterior capsule opacification. The clouding may develop months or years after the initial cataract surgery.

Treating a secondary cataract involves YAG laser capsulotomy. The word capsulotomy means "cutting into the capsule." YAG is an acronym for yttrium, aluminum and garnet, the name of the device used for the procedure. In this technique, the special laser creates a small opening in the clouded capsule membrane that allows light to pass through.

Laser capsulotomy is a quick, painless outpatient procedure. After the procedure, you may need to remain in your doctor's office for a short time to make sure your eye pressure isn't elevated. In some people, particularly those who have glaucoma or are extremely nearsighted, YAG laser capsulotomy can increase eye pressure. Other complications are rare but can include swelling of the macula and detachment of the retina.

- Gritty sensation or the feeling of an eyelash caught in your eye
- Sensitivity to light and wind

Expect to use eye drops for several weeks after cataract surgery to prevent infection, treat inflammation and help control eye pressure. After several days, the discomfort in your eye should begin to diminish.

You can help protect the eye by wearing glasses or an eye patch during the day and an eye shield at night until your eye doctor advises otherwise.

After surgery, don't:
- Bump your eye. Move slowly and carefully, especially on stairs.
- Rub your eye. This could cause problems at the surgical site and possibly prevent proper healing.
- Drive. Avoid driving until your doctor advises you to do so.
- Exercise strenuously the first couple of weeks to ensure proper healing. Your doctor can recommend when you may resume these activities.
- Expose yourself to dirty, dusty environments for a few weeks. This could irritate your eye and delay healing.

You may:
- Read, watch TV, and look at a cellphone or computer screen to the degree that's comfortable to you
- Bend down to tie your shoes
- Bathe or shower during the first week, but avoid getting water directly into the affected eye
- Walk
- Drive, once your doctor says it's OK

Contact your doctor immediately if any of these signs and symptoms occur:
- Worsening of your vision
- Persistent pain despite use of pain medications
- A significant increase in eye redness or secretions from the eye
- Light flashes or multiple new spots (floaters) in your field of vision
- Nausea, vomiting or excessive coughing

Whether you'll need eyeglasses after surgery may depend on which type of intraocular lens is implanted (see "Intraocular lens options" on page 118). With a multifocal lens, you may have sharp focus at a variety of distances without use of corrective lenses. With a monofocal lens, you'll likely see distant objects clearly but may need reading glasses.

Astigmatism after cataract surgery is less of a problem thanks to precision technology. After surgery, when your eyes have healed, your eye doctor can assess whether corrective lenses are needed.

Complications from cataract surgery are rare, and the problems are usually treatable. They include inflammation, infection, bleeding and swelling. The risk of complications is greater for people with other eye diseases or serious medical problems.

Occasionally, cataract surgery fails to improve vision. This is often because of a preexisting eye condition, such as glaucoma or macular degeneration. It may be necessary to treat these eye problems before proceeding with cataract surgery.

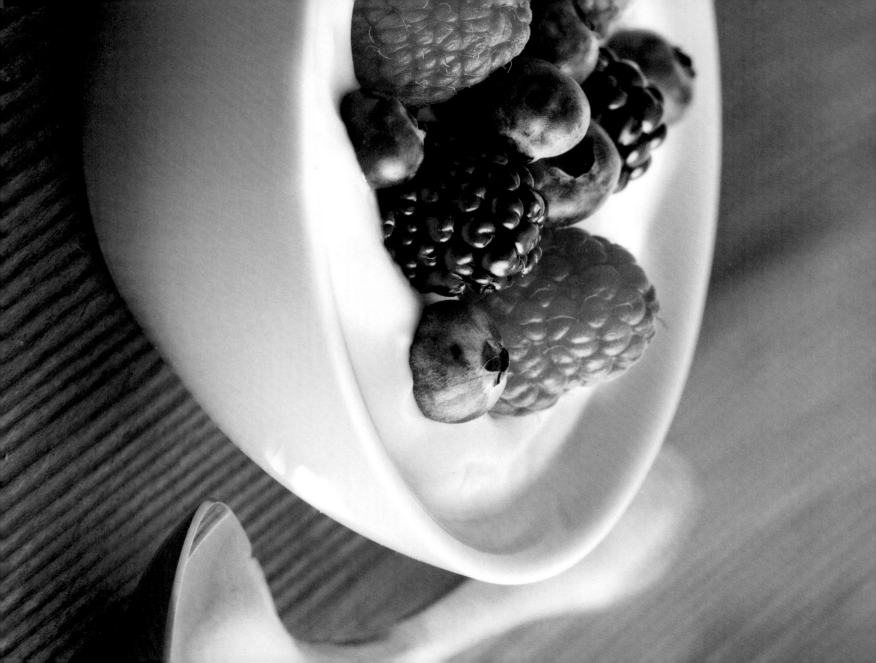

PREVENTION

Most cataracts occur naturally with age, and they can't be avoided. But you may be able to slow cataract progression. Here are some steps that may slow or possibly even prevent the development of a cataract:

- **Don't smoke.** Smoking produces the unstable molecules known as free radicals, which increase your risk of cataracts.

- **Eat a healthy, balanced diet.** Try to include plenty of fruits and vegetables in your diet. Research suggests that antioxidants in these foods may slow the development of cataracts.

- **Use sun protection.** Ultraviolet (UV) light may assist the development of cataracts. Wear sunglasses outdoors that block UVA and UVB radiation.

- **Take care of other health problems.** Follow your treatment plan if you have diabetes or other medical conditions that can increase your risk of developing a cataract.

Researchers continue to explore new ways to treat and possibly prevent cataracts. In the meantime, chances are excellent that cataract surgery can fully restore your vision, provided you have no other eye conditions.

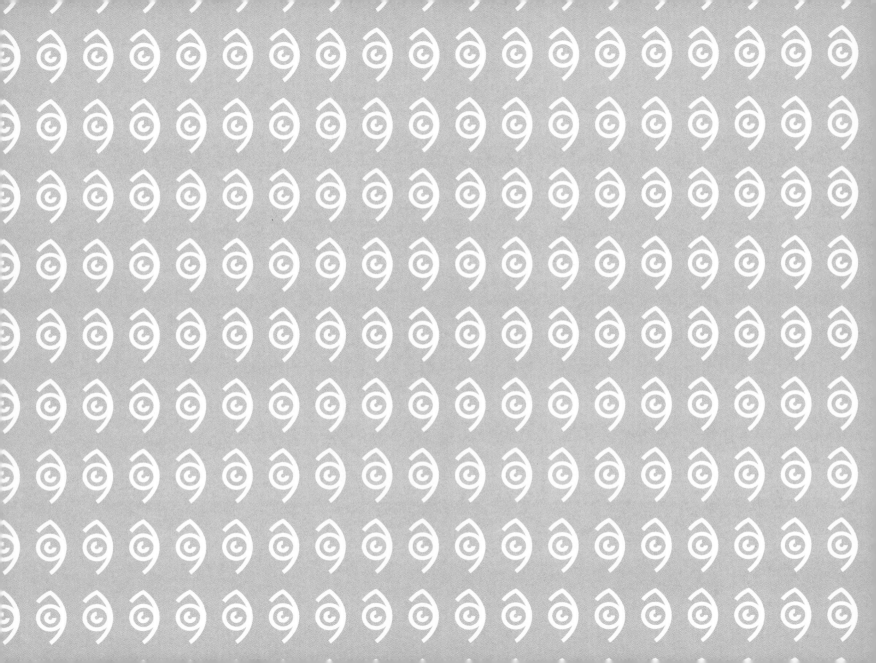

7

Common eye conditions

Your eyes are complex organs with many delicate parts and sensitive functions. Most of the time — with or without the help of corrective lenses — your eyes provide dependable vision. But there's plenty of opportunity for problems that may affect your vision, whether due to an injury, infection, allergic reaction, general wear and tear, or age-related changes.

Many common eye conditions are troublesome. Your eyes may become red, itchy, irritated or dry. Your eyelids may twitch, swell or sag. Your tear ducts may produce too much fluid or too little fluid. Any of these problems can affect your ability to see clearly — and often you may have more than one problem to worry about. As distressing as they can be, these conditions typically don't damage your sight permanently.

Anytime you notice that your vision is impaired, it's good to consult an eye doctor, even if the symptoms seem minor. A serious eye problem isn't always immediately obvious, and delay in seeing a doctor may allow damage to worsen and potentially become permanent.

Some of the most common eye problems are described in this section, along with their treatment. With proper care — having consulted your eye doctor and heeding his or her advice — you should be able to ease the symptoms and regain clear vision.

For the most part, all of the conditions described in this section may be treated at home. It's important that you follow recommendations for care and take steps to prevent a recurrence.

PAINFUL, ITCHY OR IRRITATED EYES

Several conditions can cause eye pain or discomfort. Following are some of the more common.

Pink eye (conjunctivitis)

The sudden onset of pink or red coloration in an eye, especially if it's accompanied by irritation and tearing, may signal an inflammation known as conjunctivitis, commonly called pink eye.

Conjunctivitis may be caused by a virus, bacterium or allergic reaction. Viral and bacterial conjunctivitis are extremely infectious and are often associated with

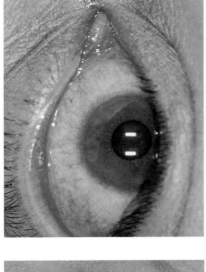

VIRAL CONJUNCTIVITIS

Viral infection of the eye enlarges blood vessels in the conjunctiva, giving it a swollen, red and teary appearance.

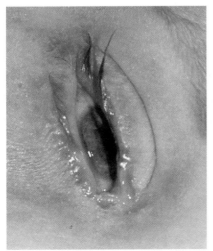

a cold or sore throat. Allergic conjunctivitis stems from exposure to an allergen, a substance that irritates the eye.

All forms of conjunctivitis have symptoms in common. Inflammation enlarges the small blood vessels of the clear, resilient membrane that lines the eye (conjunctiva), giving it a reddish or pinkish coloration.

Your eye may also become itchy and teary. You may feel a scratchy sensation when you blink, as if fine grains of sand were lodged under the eyelids. You may wake up in the morning with your eyelids encrusted with discharge. You may have

BACTERIAL CONJUNCTIVITIS

Bacterial conjunctivitis causes redness and swelling similar to the viral form but also typically develops a mucous discharge that's thicker than the one produced by viral conjunctivitis.

blurred vision and be overly sensitive to light. If you wear contacts, you need to stop wearing them as soon as signs and symptoms appear.

Applying a wet compress may soothe discomfort in the affected eye. A warm compress works best for viral and bacterial conjunctivitis, but a cold compress helps relieve the itching of allergic conjunctivitis. Soak a clean cloth in water, squeeze it dry and lay it over your closed eyelids for 10 minutes.

If your symptoms don't start to get better within a day or two, make an appointment with your eye doctor or a medical provider to make sure that you don't have a more serious eye infection or eye condition. If, in addition to redness, you experience eye pain or a feeling that something is stuck in your eye (foreign body sensation), seek urgent care.

Bacterial conjunctivitis

Along with irritation, bacterial conjunctivitis produces a sticky, yellow-green discharge that's thicker than the discharge from viral conjunctivitis. When you wake up in the morning, your eyes may be matted shut by crusty discharge. The infection often starts in one eye and spreads to the other.

The bacteria that cause conjunctivitis can be encountered from many sources, including another person with a bacterial infection. Germs are passed from person to person through infected body fluids or by hand-to-eye contact. Wearing contact lenses that aren't cleaned properly also can cause bacterial conjunctivitis.

Eye drops or ointment prescribed by your doctor can help treat bacterial conjunctivitis, but there's no such treatment for the viral form.

Viral conjunctivitis

Viral conjunctivitis spreads through contact with contaminated tears or nasal fluids. Signs and symptoms of viral conjunctivitis usually appear 7 to 10 days after you've been infected. The condition produces a watery or mucous discharge. Often, an infection in one eye leads to an infection in the other eye.

Unfortunately, there's really nothing that you can do to treat viral conjunctivitis. You must wait for the infection to run its course and go away on its own — which can take up to a couple of weeks.

Allergic conjunctivitis

Unlike viral and bacterial conjunctivitis, which are caused by infection, allergic conjunctivitis is your body's response to an allergen — a substance that irritates the eye. Your body reacts by releasing chemicals, such as histamine, that cause the allergy symptoms.

Common allergens include pollen, dust, mold, animal dander and skin, chemicals in common household products, spray perfumes, and certain kinds of medications. A substance that may be highly allergenic to you may have little or no effect on someone else.

Allergic conjunctivitis, like the viral and bacterial forms, can make your eyes red and itchy. A ropy discharge may form, particularly after rubbing your eyes. Other symptoms may include intense tearing, a runny nose and sneezing. The condition often affects both eyes at the same time.

Depending on the allergic trigger, treatment may clear up the inflammation quickly or it may only ease the discomfort. For example, conjunctivitis associated with hay fever can last the whole season and return every year.

Eye drops and oral medications that may help relieve allergy symptoms include:

• **Decongestants.** They contain chemicals that reduce eye redness and relieve nasal congestion. Most are available without a prescription and some are combined with an antihistamine. Prolonged use may have a rebound effect, causing increased eye swelling and redness. Don't use decongestant eye drops if you have glaucoma.

• **Antihistamines.** Antihistamines block the action of histamine, the chemical released by your immune system that's responsible for many allergy symptoms. Antihistamines are available by prescription or over the counter.

• **Nonsteroidal anti-inflammatory drugs (NSAIDs).** They include medications such as ibuprofen (Advil, Motrin IB) and naproxen sodium (Aleve) that help relieve inflammation and swelling.

• **Mast cell stabilizers.** These medications reduce the action of mast cells that release histamine and other chemicals causing allergy symptoms. The drugs function best when they're used before you're exposed to the allergen. Some eye drops combine antihistamine and mast cell stabilizers.

• **Corticosteroid eye drops.** Corticosteroids may be prescribed if antihistamine and decongestant medications fail to relieve symptoms. These potent medications should only be used as prescribed by your eye doctor because prolonged use can increase your risk of glaucoma, cataracts and eye infections.

STOPPING THE SPREAD

Good hygiene is essential for preventing the spread of conjunctivitis.

• Don't allow your hands to touch the area around your eyes.
• Wash your hands frequently.
• Dispose of facial tissues immediately after use.
• Don't share towels, washcloths, pillowcases, handkerchiefs, contact lenses, lens-cleaning solution or eye drops with another person.
• Stay home from work, school or social activities until you have no discharge from your eyes.
• Dispose of mascara, and purchase new when the infection is gone.

Perhaps the best way to deal with allergic conjunctivitis is to strictly avoid the allergens that trigger your symptoms — although that's not always easy to do. If you're allergic to pollen, for example, and pollen counts in the air are high, try to stay indoors, keep your doors and windows closed, and use an air conditioner. If you're allergic to animal dander, you may need to avoid pets that shed hair. If a chemical in your contact lens solution causes a reaction, try switching brands or wear glasses.

Other reactions

Some allergic reactions can be a source of discomfort without necessarily reddening the eye. This type of reaction may be due to substances that are not true allergens, such as cigarette smoke, perfume and exhaust fumes. Your eyes may become irritated, itchy and watery. Your eyelids may become puffy. Dark circles may appear under your eyes, and scaly, red skin may appear around your eyes. You may be tempted to rub your eyes, but doing so just causes more irritation.

Treatment for this type of reaction is the same as that for allergic conjunctivitis. For many people, an antihistamine provides sufficient relief. Applying a cold compress several times a day may decrease swelling around your eyes. In severe cases, your doctor may prescribe medication, such as a steroid cream or ointment. Applying a steroid near the eyes involves risk, so it's important to use the medication exactly as prescribed.

Scleritis and episcleritis

The sclera is the layer of tissue that forms the wall of your eyeball. Sandwiched between the sclera and the outer membrane (conjunctiva) is a transparent tissue called the episclera. Occasionally, the sclera or episclera becomes inflamed.

Symptoms include patchy redness and swelling in the eye. Episcleritis is a mild inflammation that generally disappears on its own after a week or two. Scleritis is a less common but more serious disorder, which may be associated with inflammatory bowel disease or rheumatoid arthritis. It may be accompanied by dull pain and blurred vision. Steroids in drop or ointment form may help reduce inflammation. Oral anti-inflammatory drugs also may be used.

Uveitis

The uvea is a middle layer of tissue in the wall of the eye, which includes the choroid, iris and ciliary body. Inflammation of the uvea is called uveitis. When the inflammation affects primarily the iris, the condition is known as iritis. Symptoms may appear suddenly — including eye pain and redness, blurred vision, floaters, sensitivity to light, and decreased vision — and they may get worse quickly.

The condition may be associated with disorders such as rheumatoid arthritis or inflammatory bowel disease, infections such as syphilis or tuberculosis, eye injury, and certain cancers. Sometimes, the cause is unknown. Untreated, uveitis can permanently damage the eye. Besides vision loss, complications may include glaucoma, cataract, and retinal and optic nerve damage.

Your eye doctor may treat uveitis with anti-inflammatory drugs, such as corticosteroids, often in eye drop form. Steroids may be prescribed orally or as injections for more-severe cases. If the condition is caused by infection, antibiotics may be prescribed. If the uveitis is caused by an underlying condition, treatment will focus on correcting or managing that condition.

Eye scratch

The cornea is the most exposed surface of the eye and susceptible to injury. An abrasion can occur when small particles of dirt, sand, wood or metal come in contact with the cornea, or if you wear your contact lenses for too long.

Following injury, the tissue around your eye may swell and the eye itself may redden and hurt intensely. You may blink more than usual. Some people don't feel symptoms for hours, then find themselves in extreme discomfort later.

Simple corneal abrasions are treated first by removing the foreign material. Try rinsing your eye with clean water or a saline solution. Don't rub the eye, and don't touch the eye surface with cotton swabs or tweezers, which may only make the abrasion worse. Allow the eye time to heal itself, which may take a couple of

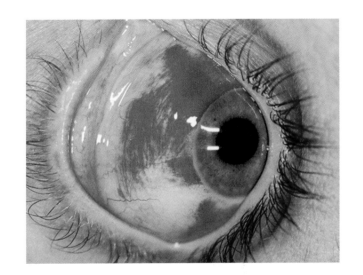

days. Your eye doctor may apply an antibiotic to prevent infection and prescribe a pain reliever. More serious injury to the cornea sometimes requires surgical treatment.

Subconjunctival hemorrhage

Looking in a mirror and seeing a bright red patch on the white (sclera) of your eye

SUBCONJUNCTIVAL HEMORRHAGE

It occurs when a small blood vessel in the eye breaks. The condition may look scary, but it's harmless and usually disappears in a few days.

can be alarming. This condition is usually caused by bleeding (hemorrhage) from a broken blood vessel in the conjunctiva. It may occur after you've coughed, sneezed or vomited forcefully. Trauma to the eye also may cause bleeding. Often, there's no identifiable cause.

The condition should improve on its own. If the hemorrhage is painful or you get them recurrently, see your eye doctor.

EYELID-RELATED PROBLEMS

Several different conditions can affect your eyelids, producing a variety of signs and symptoms.

Sty

A sty is a red lump near the edge of your eyelid that may look like a boil or pimple. It's caused by a bacterial infection around the root of an eyelash. A sty is usually harmless, but as it fills with pus it can become painful when touched.

With a sty, the swelling on your eyelid develops gradually over several days. About a week after it first appears, the sty usually ruptures, which relieves the pain. The swelling will go down in another week or so. You may get more than one sty because the bacteria can spread and infect other eyelash follicles.

As tempting as it may be, don't try to pop the sty or squeeze pus from it because doing so may allow the infection to spread. Let the sty burst on its own. Once it has opened, wash your eyelid thoroughly to prevent the bacteria from spreading.

To help relieve pain, place a warm washcloth or compress over your closed eyes. Apply the compress for 10 or 15 minutes at a time. Doing this several times a day may encourage the sty to drain on its own.

Consult your eye doctor if the sty interferes with your vision, if it doesn't disappear on its own or if redness and swelling involve the entire eyelid or extend to your cheek or other parts of your face.

A stubborn sty may need to be lanced and drained. If you're prone to recurring sties, your doctor may prescribe antibiotic treatment.

STY

A sty is a painful red lump caused by a bacterial infection around the root of an eyelash that is usually harmless.

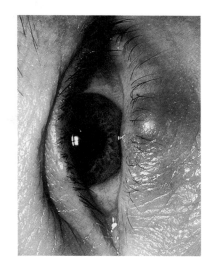

Chalazion

Another form of swelling on the eyelid is a chalazion. Unlike a sty, the swelling is relatively painless and develops away from the eyelid edge. A chalazion is not an infection. It's caused by the blockage of a small oil gland in the eyelid. Chalazions often start out very small but may grow to the size of a pea.

A chalazion typically goes away without treatment, although how long that takes may vary from several weeks to a couple of months. Apply a warm compress to the area four times a day for 10 to 15 minutes to encourage healing. You also can massage the area to try to break up the lump.

If the chalazion gets big enough to affect your vision, your doctor may prescribe an antibiotic ointment. If this treatment is unsuccessful or if the swelling continues to enlarge, the chalazion may need to be drained surgically.

Blepharitis

Blepharitis is an inflammation of the eyelids along the lid margins where the eyelashes grow. The condition often occurs when tiny oil glands located near the base of the eyelashes malfunction. Oil buildup at the glands encourages the growth of bacteria, which irritates the eyelids (see the photo on the opposite page). Although blepharitis may feel unattractive, it doesn't permanently damage your eyesight.

Signs and symptoms of blepharitis include itchy, burning or swollen eyelids, watery or red eyes, a gritty sensation in the eyes, sensitivity to light, frothy tears, and flaking skin around the eyes.

The eyelids appear greasy and crusted with scales that cling to the lashes and cause the eyelids to stick together at night. Don't be too concerned if you have to pry your eyes open in the morning because of the sticky secretions. You may also notice dried tear secretions around your eyes in the morning that feel like small grains of sand.

Blepharitis may stem from factors other than malfunctioning oil glands. Condi-

CHALAZION

A chalazion (on the upper eyelid) is a relatively painless lump caused by the blockage of an oil gland, usually located away from the eyelid edge. (A sty is located on the lower eyelid.)

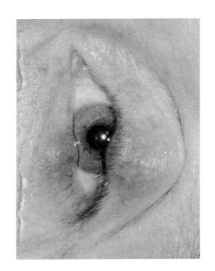

tions associated with blepharitis include dandruff of the scalp and eyebrows (seborrheic dermatitis) and a skin condition characterized by facial redness (rosacea). Possible complications of blepharitis include the loss of eyelashes, abnormal eyelash growth, development of a sty or chalazion, excess tearing or dry eyes, chronic pink eye, and injury to the cornea.

Blepharitis is often a chronic condition that can be difficult to treat. The key is good hygiene that allows you to help control the symptoms. Follow this remedy once or twice a day:

1. Apply a warm compress over your closed eyes for approximately 10 minutes to loosen the crusty deposits on your eyelids.

2. Immediately after the compress, use a washcloth moistened with warm water and a few drops of baby shampoo to wash away oily debris at the base of your eyelashes. To do this, gently pull each eyelid away from your eye to avoid accidental injury to your cornea from the motions of your washcloth.

3. Rinse your eyelids with warm water and gently pat them dry with a clean, dry towel.

Ask your doctor about using a topical antibacterial solution after cleaning your eyelids. Continue daily cleanings until your symptoms disappear. Although you may be able to decrease the frequency of cleaning, you'll want to maintain an eyelid care routine to prevent a recurrence.

BLEPHARITIS

An eyelid with blepharitis may appear red and swollen with scaly, greasy debris along the lid margin. Blepharitis is often associated with dandruff of the scalp and the eyebrows.

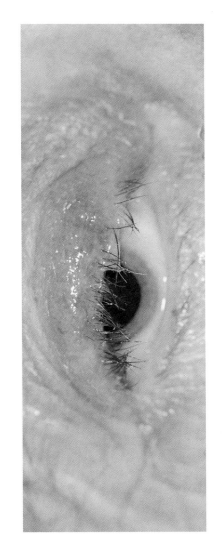

If the blepharitis doesn't improve with regular cleaning, contact your doctor. He or she may prescribe an antibiotic cream or ointment. In severe cases, eye drops containing antibiotics and corticosteroids may be prescribed.

Twitchy eyelids

From time to time your eyelid may take on a life of its own. The involuntary twitching usually lasts only for a few seconds, but it can recur. It can make you wonder if there's something wrong with your eye.

An eyelid twitch is usually considered harmless. It typically occurs on the upper lid and is similar to the occasional muscle twitch in a hand, forearm, leg or foot. No one knows exactly what causes these flutters, although they often seem to happen in times of fatigue or stress. Bright lights, caffeine and alcohol also may trigger twitchy eyelids.

Very rarely, a twitching eyelid is a symptom of a muscle or nerve disease, but this type of fluctuation tends to be distinct from the common eye twitch.

You may be able to relieve the twitching by gently massaging the affected eyelid. To do this, move your index finger back and forth from the inner to the outer part of your lid for approximately one minute. Use the same amount of pressure that you put on a computer keyboard. Massage may be more effective if you use a warm compress on your eyelid for about 10 minutes beforehand.

Itchy eyelids

Itchiness around your eyes often accompanies seasonal allergies, but it may also indicate contact dermatitis. This inflammation is a result of your fingers coming in contact with an irritating substance and then touching your eyelids. Cosmetics also may cause allergic reactions to the sensitive skin around your eyes.

If your eyelids itch, don't rub or scratch them excessively. Rubbing ultimately can cause eczema, with persistent itching and scaling. If your eyelids are sensitive to certain cosmetics or other materials, avoid using them.

Entropion and ectropion

Sometimes, an eyelid (usually a lower lid) turns in toward the eye, allowing the eyelid and eyelashes to rub against the eye's surface. This condition is called entropion. In addition to irritation, entropion causes tearing, redness, discharge, crusting of the eyelid and a feeling that something is lodged in the eye. In severe cases, the turned-in lashes may scratch the cornea, causing an infection.

Most often, entropion develops when eyelid tissue weakens due to aging. An early sign of the condition is eye irritation in the morning, which usually clears during the day. The irritation often becomes more frequent, even constant.

Ectropion describes the sagging and turning out of the eyelid (usually a lower lid). As a result, your eyelids can no longer close properly. Without adequate protection, the exposed surface of the eye becomes dry and inflamed. Tears pool in the corners of the eyes and overflow onto the eyelids. Rubbing the eye leads to further irritation.

Like entropion, ectropion is most often a result of the age-related weakening of eyelid tissue. The condition may also stem from a facial nerve disorder, trauma, tumors or previous eyelid surgery. Sometimes, it may be associated with an underlying condition such as atopic dermatitis or lupus. Untreated ectropion may lead to eye infection and corneal damage.

Artificial tears or eye ointments can help keep the cornea lubricated and offer temporary relief from irritation. Some people wear an eye shield at night to retain moisture in the eye. Other people apply a transparent adhesive tape (skin tape) on the eyelid and along the sides of the eye to help hold the lid in place when sleeping at night.

The primary means of treating entropion and ectropion is surgery to reposition the eyelids. This often involves removing a small section of tissue from the eyelid, which serves to tighten the tendons and muscles of the lid. This simple procedure is performed on an outpatient basis using local anesthetic. After surgery, you may

ENTROPION AND ECTROPION

With entropion (left) the eyelid turns inward, allowing the lashes to rub against and irritate the eyeball. With ectropion (right) the eyelid sags away from the eyeball. Lacking protection and sufficient lubrication, the eye becomes red and irritated.

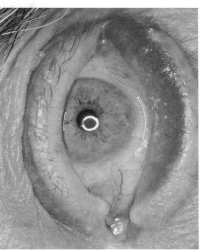

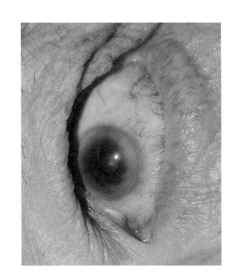

wear an eye patch overnight and apply antibiotic ointment to the area for about a week.

If you can't tolerate surgery or you have to delay it, other options may be considered. They include:

- **Soft contact lens.** Your eye doctor may suggest that you use a type of soft contact lens as a sort of corneal bandage to help ease symptoms. These are available with or without a refractive prescription.

- **Botox.** With this treatment, small amounts of OnabotulinumtoxinA (Botox) injected into the lower eyelid can turn the eyelid out. You may get a series of injections, with effects lasting up to six months.

- **Stitches that turn the eyelid outward.** This procedure can be done in your doctor's office with local anesthesia. Several stitches are placed in specific locations along the affected eyelid. The stitches turn the eyelid outward, and resulting scar tissue keeps the eyelid in position even after the stitches are removed. After several months, your eyelid may turn itself back inward, so this technique isn't a long-term solution.

- **Skin tape.** Special transparent skin tape can be applied to your eyelid to keep it from turning in.

Dermatochalasis

With age, the skin of your eyelid may stretch and sag due to the accumulation of fat and the loss of muscle elasticity. This condition is called dermatochalasis, and it usually affects both eyes at the same time.

Occasionally, the skin of your upper eyelids may sag over your eyelashes to impair your side (peripheral) vision or prevent your eyes from opening completely. The lower eyelids may form what are commonly known as bags under your eyes.

Surgery to repair droopy eyelids by removing excess skin, muscle and fat is called blepharoplasty. The procedure is generally safe and can be done on an outpatient basis. Swelling or bruising should subside within two to four weeks. Mild cases may be treated with laser surgery that tightens the tissue without removing it.

Many people express satisfaction with the results of surgery, although for some, drooping eyelids may recur. Insurance coverage may depend on whether the condition impairs vision.

Ptosis

Ptosis results from a weakness of the eye muscle controlling your upper eyelid, which is responsible for raising the lid and keeping it in an open position. Whereas dermatochalasis results in sagging eyelid skin, ptosis causes the entire eyelid to droop.

A drooping upper eyelid will reduce your field of vision. You may try to compensate for this by continually arching your eyebrows in an effort to keep the upper lid raised.

Ptosis often runs in families and can affect one or both eyes. Some children are born with the condition — usually in just one eye. In adults, ptosis may be a result of aging or injury, or a condition affecting nerve and muscle response, such as myasthenia gravis, diabetes or a brain tumor.

A drooping eyelid that develops suddenly requires immediate attention because this may be the sign of a stroke or another serious condition.

If ptosis isn't affecting your vision and you're not bothered by your appearance, your doctor may not treat the condition. But if ptosis is reducing your vision, a thorough eye examination may be necessary. Your doctor will seek out the cause of the problem, as well as determine the best course of treatment.

DERMATOCHALASIS

With dermatochalasis, the skin of the upper eyelid relaxes. The skin may droop over the eyelashes and interfere with your vision. The condition is sometimes referred to as "baggy eyes."

If the droop is due to a nerve or muscle condition, treating the underlying cause may help. If the droop is due to aging or injury, your doctor may recommend surgery to strengthen the muscle. This is a complicated procedure that should be performed by a specialist.

TEAR-RELATED PROBLEMS

Healthy eyes are covered by a thin film of tear fluid — a layer that moistens the eyes' surface without overflowing the eyelids. Tear glands that produce most of the fluid are located underneath the skin of the upper eyelids. Additional glands in the eyelids also produce components of tear fluid.

Tears reach the eye through openings in the upper eyelids. When you blink, your eyelids spread the fluid across the surface

PTOSIS

A weakened muscle that raises the upper eyelid can cause the entire lid to droop over the eye (in this case, the person's left eye).

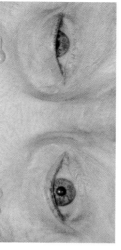

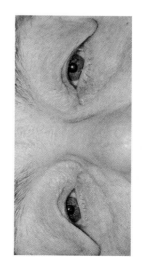

Common eye conditions   **137**

and sweep excess into tear ducts that drain to your nose — that's why your nose often runs when you cry. Basic tearing occurs at a continuous, steady rate to prevent dry eyes and maintain clear vision.

Reflex tearing produces a large amount of fluid in response to injury or strong emotion, often causing tears to overflow. For example, when your eyes are affected by smoke, extra tears form to wash away the foreign material. A sad movie or a joyous wedding also can make tears stream down your cheeks.

There are other causes of teary eyes, including allergic reactions, eye or sinus infections, and nasal problems. Occasionally, tear duct problems result in continuous tearing.

Dry eyes

Tear production tends to decrease as you get older, and decreased production destabilizes the tear film, creating dry spots on the surface that irritate the eye and reduce vision. Some people produce a normal amount of tears, but the composition of their tear fluid is of poor quality. The tears lack essential components for eye lubrication. Eyelid problems also can cause dry eyes.

The medical term for dry eyes is kerato-conjunctivitis sicca. The condition usually affects both eyes at the same time. Signs and symptoms include a stinging, burning or scratchy sensation, swelling, redness, and stringy mucus in or around the eyes.

You may also experience eye fatigue and increased sensitivity to light.

Dry eyes are associated with certain medical conditions such as rheumatoid

THE TEAR SYSTEM

The tear gland, located in the orbit above each eye, produces a continuous supply of tear fluid. The fluid is spread across the surface of your eye by the blinking action of your eyelids. A thin layer of tear fluid on the surface nourishes and lubricates your eye and washes away debris. Oil mixed into the tear solution from small glands in your eyelids helps keep the fluid from evaporating too quickly. Excess fluid is swept to ducts at the side of your eye and drains into your nose, or it overflows the lids as tears.

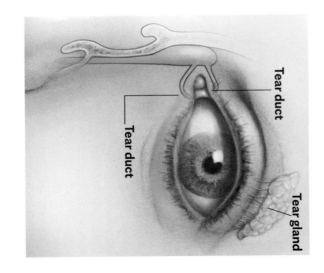

Tear duct

Tear duct

Tear gland

arthritis and Sjogren's syndrome. Dry eyes don't usually cause permanent vision damage, but the condition is uncomfortable, prompting people to seek treatment.

Tear quality

Tears are more than just water. They're a complex mixture that also includes fatty oils, proteins, electrolytes and bacteria-fighting substances. This exact mixture is necessary to keep the eye surface moist, smooth and clear.

Tear film has three basic layers:

- **Mucus.** The inner layer consists of mucus, which allows tears to spread evenly across the surface.
- **Water.** The middle layer is mostly water with a little bit of salt. It cleanses the eye and washes away foreign irritants.
- **Oil.** The outer layer, produced by glands on the edge of the eyelid,

contains fatty oils. The oil smooths the tear film and slows the evaporation of the watery middle layer.

Sometimes, this mix of ingredients is off balance, which causes tear fluid to evaporate too fast. Certain diseases can change the oil and mucous layers of your tears. Some skin disorders can disrupt production of the oil layer. Any of these events can dry the eye's surface.

Treatment goals for dry eyes are to restore a more normal tear film and to minimize the consequences of dryness.

- **Adding tears.** A mild case of dry eyes can often be treated with artificial tears sold over the counter. Use the lubricating drops as needed to provide relief. Preservative-free eye drops work best.
- **Medications.** The medication cyclosporine (Restasis) may be prescribed to treat chronic dry eyes. It reduces inflammation on the surface of your

IF MY EYES ARE DRY, WHY ARE THEY WATERING?

It may seem like a contradiction, but it's possible to have dry eyes and still have tears streaming down your cheeks. When your eyes are irritated from dryness, the tear glands respond by flooding the eyes with reflex tears. Because reflex tears contain more water and less oil than basic tears do, they evaporate faster and don't help the dryness. Excess fluid overwhelms the tear ducts and overflows your eyelids.

If your eyes feel dry and irritated, your doctor can test the quantity and quality of your tears. With the Schirmer test, blotting strips are placed under your lower eyelids to measure how much of the strips are soaked by your tears. Other tests use eye drops with special dyes to determine the surface condition of your eye and measure the rate at which your tears evaporate.

eyes. Some people experience a burning sensation in their eyes when using the drug. Other medications that reduce eyelid inflammation, lubricate your eyes or help stimulate tear production may also be recommended.

- **Conserving tears.** This procedure involves partially or completely closing your tear ducts with tiny, removable silicone plugs that help retain fluid by keeping tears from leaving the eye too quickly. In a more permanent option, a surgeon uses heat to shrink tissue at the opening of the tear duct, causing scarring that closes the duct.

- **Special contact lenses.** Ask your eye doctor about newer contact lenses designed to help people with dry eyes. Some people with severe dry eyes may opt for special contact lenses that protect the surface of the eyes and trap moisture. These are called scleral lenses or bandage lenses.

- **Light therapy and eyelid massage.** A technique called intense-pulsed light therapy followed by massage of the eye-

lids may help some people with severe dry eyes.

Overflowing tears

Excess tear production occurs mostly among older adults and is associated with aging or injury to the nose. Too much tearing may also result from an eye abrasion, eyelid infection, inward-growing eyelashes, allergies or nasal problems. When this happens, tear fluid backs up and spills over your eyelid, causing tears to run down your cheeks.

Excessive tearing can also result from inadequate drainage through the tear ducts. A tear duct can become blocked by infection or by small particles of dirt or loose skin cells lodged in the duct.

See your doctor if tears constantly flow over a period of several days. If the problem is a blocked duct, he or she may flush (irrigate) the tear duct in a simple outpatient procedure.

PRESERVING MOISTURE

Like any kind of liquid, tear fluid evaporates when it's exposed to air. Here are some simple steps to slow the evaporation:

- Avoid air blowing in your eyes from hair dryers, air conditioners or fans.
- Wear eyeglasses on windy days and goggles while swimming.
- Keep your home humidity between 30% and 50%. In the winter, a humidifier will add moisture to indoor air.
- Avoid rubbing your eyes, which may cause further irritation.
- Remember to blink. Blinking helps spread fluid more evenly.
- Avoid smoke, which can worsen dry eyes symptoms.
- Use artificial tears regularly to keep your eyes well lubricated.

Infected tear duct

Occasionally, a tear duct can become infected from bacteria that has collected in stagnant tears. This condition is called dacryocystitis. When it happens, the tissue between your eye and the bridge of your nose becomes swollen, red and tender. Tears can no longer drain into your nose, causing an excessive amount of tearing.

Your doctor may prescribe an antibiotic for the infection. Applying a warm compress to the eye several times a day may help relieve discomfort.

If the symptoms are severe and don't improve with medication, your eye doctor may recommend surgery to create a new tear duct. Thin silicone tubing is used to keep the new duct open while healing occurs. In rare cases, it's necessary to surgically implant an artificial tear duct. The artificial duct is made of unbreakable glass.

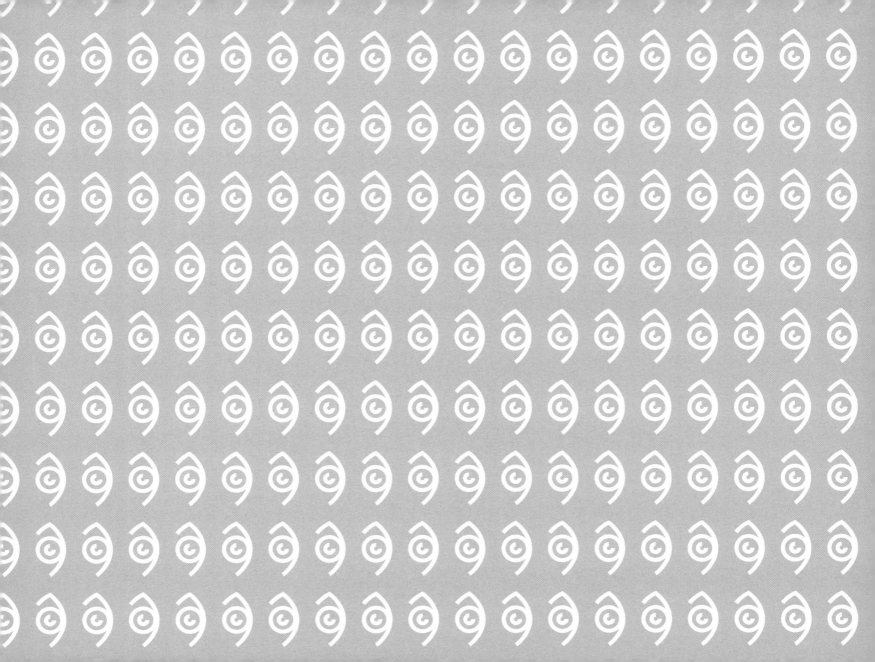

Eye conditions affecting children

Childhood is an important time for vision development. As a child grows, the eyes become better at many functions, including quickly shifting focus between near and far distances, seeing 3D objects, and focusing on and following moving objects.

A child's vision is developing up until about age 10, and these early years set the stage for vision health later in life.

During childhood, connections are established between the eyes and the brain. The brain relies on the retina — the thin, light-sensitive tissue at the back of the eye — to ensure that these connections develop properly and that clear images are transmitted. Sometimes, problems can interfere with this process, threatening a child's ability to see.

Vision problems in children range from minor to serious and even life-threatening. This chapter covers common and uncommon eye diseases. The terms *congenital* and *acquired* are used on occasion. Congenital conditions are those that children are born with or that appear very soon after birth. Acquired conditions are conditions that develop after birth or later during childhood.

The terms *recessive* and *dominant* may be used when discussing eye disorders that are inherited or are associated with changes to genes (genetic mutations). An eye disease inherited through a recessive gene mutation means that both parents carry an abnormal copy of a gene, and each parent passes along a copy to the child. A dominant gene mutation requires only one parent to pass along an abnormal

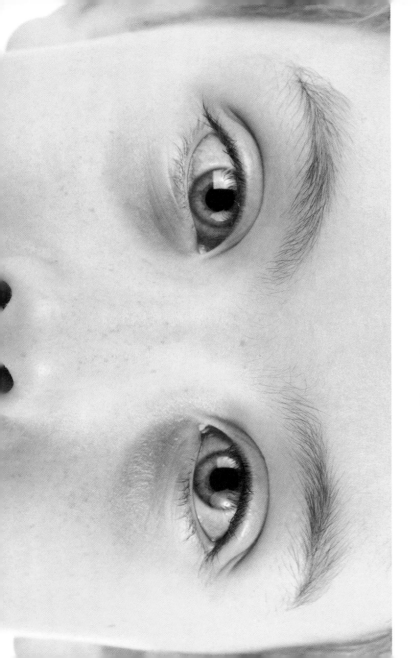

gene for a child to develop a disease. Sometimes, genes are only passed along from a mother to a child — usually a son — referred to as an X-chromosome-linked disorder. It's important to note that having parents who carry a genetic mutation doesn't guarantee a child will develop the condition.

COMMON VISION PROBLEMS

Children tend not to complain about difficulties seeing, but many times the signs — both obvious and more subtle — are there. A parent may suspect something is wrong when a child squints while watching television or turns his or her head to observe something. Less obvious, children with vision problems may frequently lose their place while reading or may lose interest in any activity that requires them to use their eyes for lengthy periods. Some children may turn their heads to get a better look at something that's right in front of them.

Because parents are often the first to be aware of vision problems in their children, it's important to bring up any concerns to your child's health care provider. Certain vision problems are relatively common among children. For example, amblyopia is the most common cause of decreased sight in childhood, occurring in up to 4% of children.

Pink eye (conjunctivitis)

Conjunctivitis is an inflammation or infection in the transparent membrane (conjunctiva) that lines the eyelid and covers the white part of the eyeball. When small blood vessels in the conjunctiva become inflamed, they're more visible, which is what causes the whites of the eyes to appear reddish or pink. In addition to redness, other signs and symptoms include itchiness, a gritty feeling, a discharge that forms a crust, and tearing in one or both eyes. Though pink eye can be irritating, it rarely affects vision.

Common causes of pink eye are viruses, bacteria and allergic reactions. Viral and bacterial conjunctivitis can occur along with colds or symptoms of a respiratory infection. Newborns are susceptible to a severe form of pink eye known as ophthalmia neonatorum. This infection occurs when a baby's eyes get exposed to bacteria naturally present in the birth canal. The condition needs to be treated with an antibiotic ointment immediately to prevent vision loss.

In most cases, a child doesn't need eye drops. Since conjunctivitis is usually viral, antibiotic eye drops won't help. They may even cause harm by producing a medication reaction or by making the medication less effective in the future. Instead, the virus needs time to run its course, which can take a couple of weeks.

If pink eye is due to allergic conjunctivitis, your child's doctor may recommend medication to help control allergic reactions.

Treatment for pink eye is usually focused on symptom relief. Using artificial tears, cleaning the eyelids with a wet cloth, and applying cold or warm compresses several times daily may help alleviate symptoms.

In general, children are contagious as long as they're experiencing tearing or

matted eyes. Signs and symptoms usually improve within 3 to 7 days. However, it's not uncommon for the condition to spread from one eye to the other. Generally, once the tearing and matted eyes have cleared, it's OK for a child to return to school or child care.

Sometimes pink eye can cause inflammation in the cornea, which can affect vision. If a child is experiencing vision problems, eye pain, a feeling that something is stuck in the eye or light sensitivity, he or she should see a doctor.

Scratched cornea

In the front of the eye is the clear, dome-shaped cornea. Sometimes, eye trauma and foreign objects can cause a scratch (corneal abrasion) on the cornea's outer layer (epithelium). These injuries are common. In older children or adolescents, wearing contact lenses improperly can also be the culprit.

The cornea contains many nerves that relay pain messages to the brain, so severe pain and a feeling that something is in the eye are common symptoms of a corneal scratch. The affected eye may also be sensitive to light.

Most abrasions don't require treatment. Depending on the size of the abrasion and the cornea's health, its outer layer may heal over in a day or two. However, since it isn't always clear what may have caused a corneal scratch in a child, it may be a good idea to see a health care provider. If a foreign object caused a

Other conditions that can cause excessive tearing include:

- **Uveitis.** This is an inflammation of the colored part of the eye (iris). It can occur after trauma and with certain conditions, such as lupus, Kawasaki syndrome, and some forms of juvenile arthritis. In addition to watery eyes, a child with uveitis may experience light sensitivity, deep eye pain and redness of the eye. The symptoms may come on suddenly or gradually. Treatment typically involves anti-inflammatory medications and medications called cycloplegic agents.

- **Eyelid defects.** These can include conditions in which the eyelids turn inward (entropion) or they have an extra fold of skin on the lower lid (epiblepharon) that can cause tearing, redness and the feeling that something is in the eye. Most children outgrow epiblepharon by the age of 3. Significant problems may require surgery. Eyelids that become inflamed also can cause tearing, burning, itching and crusting (blepharitis).

- **Glaucoma, pink eye and corneal abrasions.** These conditions also cause tearing.

Nearsightedness, farsightedness and astigmatism

Nearsightedness (myopia), farsightedness (hyperopia) and astigmatism are common refractive errors.

Refraction is the bending of light rays as they pass from one transparent substance to another. In a normal eye, light reflect-

---

scratch, a health care provider can check to make sure the object is no longer in the eye or safely remove it if it is.

When a corneal abrasion is extensive, antibiotic drops or ointment may be prescribed to prevent infection. Wearing an eye patch over the affected eye while it heals may also be necessary. Sometimes, the eye's outer layer (epithelium) doesn't heal correctly. If this occurs, additional medical care may be needed.

Teary eyes

Tears help keep the eyes' surface moist, and they flush away debris and bacteria. The tear ducts don't produce tears; rather, they carry them away, similar to how a storm drain carries away rainwater.

Tears normally drain into the nose through tiny openings (puncta) in the inner portion of the eyes near the nose. In babies, the tear duct may not be fully open and functioning. This is the most common cause of teary eyes in infants. There may also be frequent crusting in the eyelashes, redness in the eye and a large, painful red bump over the tear duct (dacryocystitis).

Most blocked tear ducts clear up on their own in the first year of life. Those that don't can be treated with various therapies, including tear duct massage and tear duct probing. Probing uses special instruments to gradually widen the tear ducts. Sometimes a tube (stent) is placed to help with drainage and prevent a duct from becoming blocked again.

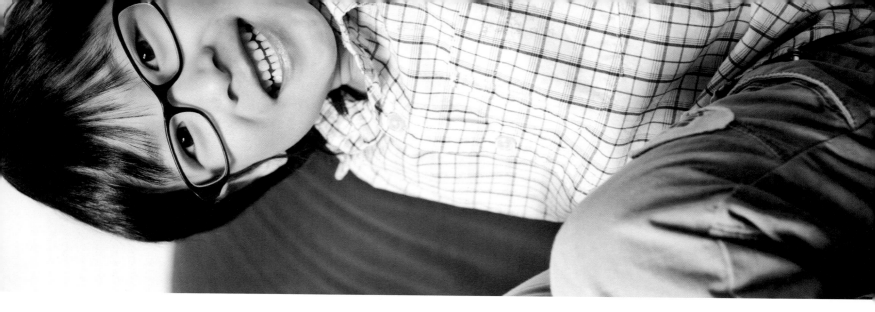

ed from an object is refracted by the cornea and lens, then focused directly on the retina. With a refractive error, the point of focus occurs just before or just behind the retina, causing blurriness.

Eyeglasses or contact lenses are the common treatment for nearsightedness, farsightedness and astigmatism. Mild cases of refractive errors may not require any treatment. In rare cases when a refractive error is accompanied by another eye condition, surgery may be necessary.

Nearsightedness

A child who is nearsighted has difficulty seeing objects clearly that are far away. Nearsightedness occurs when the eye is longer than usual, or the cornea is curved too steeply. Instead of being focused precisely on the retina, light focuses in front of the retina. The result is that things at a distance look blurry. Near-sightedness becomes more common throughout adolescence and tends to worsen during this time before finally stabilizing by the late teens or early 20s.

Sometimes steps may be taken to try and prevent nearsightedness from worsening or prevent it completely. They include

• **Eye drops.** Special drops that dilate the pupils (anti-muscarinic drops such as atropine) can slow nearsightedness progression.

• **Special contact lenses.** Use of rigid lenses placed on the eyes to temporarily change the shape of the cornea have been experimented with, but studies to support their use are limited and not of good quality.

- **Outdoor time.** Studies have found that spending more time outdoors can lower the risk of developing nearsightedness and slow its progression.

Farsightedness

In this condition, the eye is shorter than usual, or the cornea doesn't have enough of a curve to it, so light focuses behind the retina and causes close-up objects to look blurry. Severe cases may be linked to problems with visual development.

Mild farsightedness is common for infants and children. Most don't require correction because their eyes can adapt. If a child has a high degree of farsightedness, treatment is typically needed.

Astigmatism

Astigmatism means the eyeball isn't perfectly shaped like a sphere. Instead, the cornea or lens is curved more steeply in one direction than in another. As a result, the focusing power isn't consistent across the eye, and light rays aren't directed to a single point. This can make things seem a bit blurry all of the time. Astigmatism may accompany nearsightedness or farsightedness.

Amblyopia

Amblyopia refers to reduced vision in one eye — or, in rare cases, both — caused by abnormal visual development early in life. If not recognized and treated before age 9, the condition can cause permanent vision loss.

Anything that blurs a child's vision or causes the eyes to cross or turn out can result in amblyopia. In many cases, there's an imbalance in the muscles that position the eyes (strabismus amblyopia). This imbalance can cause the eyes to cross or turn out and prevents them from working in unison. The condition also may be related to a difference between the visual acuity in each eye, often due to farsightedness (refractive amblyopia). In the most-severe cases, a problem with one eye, such as a cloudy area in the lens (cataract), can prevent clear vision in that eye, reducing vision (deprivation amblyopia).

Changes to the nerve pathways between the retina and the brain cause the weaker eye to receive fewer visual signals. Eventually, the ability of both eyes to work together decreases, and the brain suppresses or ignores input from the weaker eye. As a result, the weaker eye wanders inward or outward. The condition is sometimes referred to as "lazy eye."

Premature birth, small size at birth, a family history of amblyopia and developmental disabilities can increase risk of the condition. It's crucial to treat amblyopia before age 9 when critical brain-eye connections finish developing. An interruption in this process can lead to vision loss, although sometimes treatment may be successful in older children. Treatment options depend on the cause but include:

- **Corrective eyewear.** Glasses or contacts can correct problems such as nearsightedness, farsightedness or astigmatism causing amblyopia.
- **Eye patches.** Wearing an eye patch over the unaffected eye for several hours a day can stimulate the weaker eye to work harder.
- **Bangerter filter.** A special filter is placed on the eyeglass lens of the stronger eye. The filter blurs vision in the stronger eye, like an eye patch, in an effort to stimulate and strengthen the weaker eye.
- **Eye drops.** Special eye drops can temporarily blur vision in the stronger eye and encourage a child to use the weaker eye. These may cause mild light sensitivity and eye irritation.
- **Surgery.** A child may need surgery if droopy eyelids or cataracts cause deprivation amblyopia. Surgery to straighten the eyes is an option for children whose eyes continue to cross or wander apart despite more-conservative treatment.

For most children, treatment improves vision within weeks to months. Treatment can last up to several years. Follow-up appointments are needed to monitor vision and ensure that amblyopia doesn't recur, which happens in up to 25% of children.

Strabismus

When a child's eyes don't align or look in the same direction, the condition is known as strabismus. "Crossed eyes" is a common nonmedical term for this condition.

Strabismus may occur anytime during childhood, but is more common before age 5. It may occur all of the time or only at certain times, such as when a child is tired or sick. Misaligned eyes are usually the result of problems with the brain's ability to control eye movement. Sometimes there may be a problem with the eye muscle itself.

TERMS FOR DIFFERENT TYPES

Strabismus may occur in several forms, generally described by how the eyes appear. They include the following:

- **Esotropia.** Eyes that turn inward
- **Exotropia.** Eyes that turn outward
- **Hypertropia.** Eyes that turn upward
- **Hypotropia.** Eyes that turn downward

Strabismus may occur all of the time (constant) or less frequently (intermittent). The condition may always involve the same eye (unilateral) or switch between eyes (alternating).

Eyes that turn inward tend to be the most urgent, requiring immediate attention to avoid vision damage. Eyes that turn outward are usually more intermittent and slowly progress. However, a child with any form of strabismus should see an eye specialist as soon as possible.

Depending on what type of strabismus a child has, signs and symptoms can include seeing double, closing one eye when working on something up close, tilting the head to see better, frequent headaches, problems reading, eye strain and problems seeing in bright sunlight. Misalignment also can result in amblyopia in some children.

Children most at risk for strabismus include those with neurological disorders, such as cerebral palsy, Down syndrome and brain tumors. Having severe farsightedness also can increase the risk. Sometimes, the condition may result from trauma to the brain or to nerves and muscles that help control eye movement. The condition also can run in families.

Treatment strategies include:

- **Eyeglasses or contact lenses.** Corrective eyewear may be all that's required to treat the condition, depending on the severity of the crossed eyes.
- **Vision therapy.** A specially designed program uses eye exercises to help train the brain and eyes to work better together, resulting in improved focusing and coordinated eye movements.
- **Surgery.** A procedure to reposition or shorten the length of eye muscles can realign them, so the eyes look straight. It may require more than one surgery to correct crossed eyes fully.

If diagnosed early, treatment can produce excellent results. A timely response helps preserve depth perception, decrease the chance of further drifting, and enable the eyes to function better together.

Nystagmus

Uncontrolled movement of the eyes, called nystagmus, occurs when the eyes

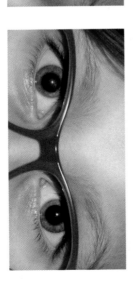

The image at left shows a child with strabismus, in which the eyes don't align. This condition is commonly referred to as crossed eyes. The image at right is of the same child, and it shows strabismus corrected with eyeglasses.

shake in back and forth, up and down, and circular directions. Movements may be fast or slow, and the condition almost always affects both eyes.

Typically, a child who has these eye movements experiences some blurriness, but the world doesn't look like it's shaking. He or she may tilt his or her head to see more clearly. Other symptoms include sensitivity to light, dizziness and problems seeing in the dark.

There are various forms of nystagmus:

Congenital nystagmus

It usually appears the first several months of life. Some children will have relatively normal vision, while others experience vision problems. In children with vision difficulties, the eyes cannot communicate with the brain about what they're seeing. This communication disruption prevents the brain from keeping the eyes steady.

Sometimes, this disconnect is due to a condition such as congenital cataracts or optic nerve hypoplasia (both explained later in this chapter). The result is an inability to sense vision, resulting in moderate to severe vision loss in both eyes.

Other children with congenital nystagmus may have nearly normal vision, but the brain lacks proper motor control for eye steadiness. This type of congenital nystagmus is more common, and its cause isn't usually known.

Acquired nystagmus

This form develops after the age of 4 months, and its causes range from brain conditions and cancer to medication side effects and genetic disorders. Because of its many causes, acquired nystagmus often requires further testing to get to the root of the problem. In most children, acquired nystagmus is spontaneous, with no family history. However, there are known genes that may cause this condition.

How a child's vision is impacted throughout his or her life depends on the type of nystagmus. A child with congenital nystagmus who develops vision problems early on and whose condition is related to an underlying condition is more likely have poor vision in future years. Children whose congenital nystagmus is related to poor motor control may have good vision.

Treatment for uncontrolled eye movements may include the following:

- **Glasses or contact lenses.** Having better vision can often help slow eye movements. Contact lenses may provide better sight compared with glasses.
- **Surgery.** Though not a standard procedure, surgery can reposition eye muscles, allowing a child with uncontrolled eye movements to see better without having to turn his or her head as much. Surgery, however, doesn't stop the eye movements.
- **Addressing the underlying cause.** In cases of acquired nystagmus, treating medical conditions or stopping a medication that's causing eye movements may eliminate them.

Ptosis

Two muscles help lift the eyelid: the levator palpebrae superioris and the Muller's muscle. When either muscle becomes weakened, an eyelid can droop in one or both eyes (ptosis). A drooping eyelid may be hereditary, it may develop as part of a more extensive syndrome, or it may occur for no known reason. The condition may be a short-term or a long-term problem, gradually worsen, or remain stable.

The most common form of eyelid drooping is congenital, and it presents during the first year of life. It generally results when the levator palpebrae superioris muscle doesn't develop normally. An acquired form of the condition occurs when the muscle weakens later in life. It's usually related to other conditions that affect the eye's muscles and nerves, such as myasthenia gravis, Horner syndrome and third cranial nerve palsy. These

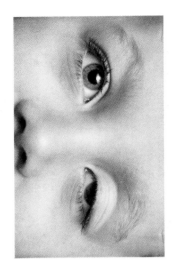

With ptosis, the upper eyelid droops over the eye. The eyelid may droop just a little or so much it covers the pupil, affecting vision.

conditions may be associated with other symptoms. For example, in addition to a drooping eyelid, Horner syndrome also causes a smaller pupil size.

Trauma and growths or tumors on the upper eyelid also can cause a drooping eyelid. In rare cases, eye deformities, extra eyelid skin, eye infections and corneal abrasions can cause an eyelid to droop.

If it doesn't affect vision, a drooping eyelid may not require treatment right away. Sometimes the condition can limit eyesight or put pressure on the eye, causing distortion and unclear vision (astigmatism). A child may hold his or her head in a "chin-up" position to better see around the droop.

When the condition interferes with vision, surgery is usually required to lift the eyelid. This may mean shortening the levator muscle or connecting the eyelid's edge to a forehead muscle. Surgery won't restore muscle function, but it can prevent vision problems and improve the eye's appearance. Potential complications of surgery include an inability for the eyelid to close correctly and dry eye.

UNCOMMON EYE CONDITIONS

Diseases such as cataracts and glaucoma generally aren't associated with children. But, uncommonly, these conditions and others can occur in infant through teenage years. Early diagnosis and treatment are often key to preserving eyesight.

Cataracts

A cataract is the clouding of the eye's lens, which either prevents light from reaching the retina or scatters it. Since light is needed to help focus images, cataracts distort images, resulting in blurry vision or blindness. Some children also will develop amblyopia.

When and how cataracts form in children varies widely. They typically present at birth when the lenses don't develop properly during pregnancy. They can also form later in childhood. Cataracts may result from genetics, eye trauma, steroid medications or diseases that affect metabolism, such as diabetes. In some instances, the cause is unknown. Some cataracts remain stable, while others worsen with time.

Not all cataracts need to be removed. Some may be very small or located away from the center of the lens, which doesn't affect vision. Frequent monitoring to make sure they don't start interfering with vision may be all that's needed.

In more-severe cases, cataracts can disrupt the important brain-eye connections formed during childhood, making it necessary to treat the condition to avoid vision loss. For most children, this means surgery to remove the cloudy lenses. In infants, severe cataracts should be removed the first weeks and months of life.

Following surgery, the eyes will need to relearn how to focus light inside the eye. Implanted lenses, special contacts or glasses can help with this:

- **Contact lenses.** In very young children, high-powered contact lenses may be placed on the eyes to help with focusing while the eyes develop. Lenses of different strengths are swapped out regularly as vision strengthens. The lenses require regular removal and cleaning.
- **Intraocular lens.** An intraocular lens is a permanent lens placed in the space where the cloudy lens was. It's generally used in children age 2 or older because of the risk of surgical complications in very young children.
- **Glasses.** Special glasses can help focus light. The lenses tend to be thick because of high magnification, so these work best for children in which both eyes are affected by cataracts.
- **Eye patch.** If a child has amblyopia because of a cataract, covering the stronger eye with a patch can strengthen the weaker eye.

The vision prognosis for children with cataracts is usually good. However, children who have cataract surgery are at increased risk of developing glaucoma.

Glaucoma

Glaucoma is the term for a group of eye diseases resulting from pressure within the eye (intraocular pressure) that's too high.

Increased eye pressure often occurs when fluid within the eye is unable to drain properly. This can eventually lead to severe vision loss, typically starting with peripheral vision and, without treatment, progressing to central vision and complete blindness.

Types of childhood glaucoma include the following:

• **Primary infantile glaucoma.** It develops in the first years of life. Infantile glaucoma results from abnormal development of eye structures, which leads to drainage problems, increased eye pressure, enlargement of the cornea and thinning of the white part of the eye (sclera). Signs and symptoms include excessive tearing, light sensitivity and a cloudy cornea, which dulls the colored part of the eye (iris).

• **Juvenile glaucoma.** This type is generally diagnosed after age 4 or 5 and develops gradually. Children usually don't have symptoms until they experience vision loss. An eye exam may pick up an enlargement of the center part of the optic nerve and elevated eye pressure. There's usually a family history of the disease, as well.

• **Secondary glaucoma.** With this type, glaucoma is a complication of another condition, including Axenfeld-Rieger syndrome, aniridia, Sturge-Weber syndrome, neurofibromatosis, tumors, chronic steroid use, trauma and surgery to remove cataracts.

Treatment for most cases of infantile glaucoma includes surgery. Procedures that create a pathway for the eye fluid to drain (such as trabeculectomy and goniotomy) are the most common. They have about an 80% to 90% success rate at controlling eye pressure when they're performed by age 2. Up to 30% of children require another procedure later on in childhood. Medication may be prescribed following surgery to help control eye pressure.

For juvenile and secondary glaucoma, eye drops and oral medications are often used. Treatments such as glasses, patches and additional surgeries can address complications from glaucoma, including nearsightedness, amblyopia and strabismus.

Preserving vision depends on many factors, including how quickly a child is treated, the type of glaucoma and the child's age. However, even with early treatment, permanent vision loss may still occur with any form of glaucoma.

Optic nerve disorders

The optic nerve is a bundle of nerve fibers that transmits visual information from the eye to the brain. The nerve's head is a round or oval disk, which is usually flat or slightly raised. In the middle of the nerve head is a depression, called the cup. Optic nerve disorders can affect any of these parts and are grouped by whether they're congenital or acquired.

Congenital optic nerve disorders typically affect the optic disk's size or shape and the nearby retina, while acquired optic nerve disorders cause cupping, swelling, or destruction of the disk.

Congenital

Certain disorders affect the nerve head. The nerve head may be missing, too small or oversized, or have an abnormal shape.

• **Hypoplasia.** It is the most common congenital disk disorder, and it typically

- involves both eyes. The disk appears to be pale and surrounded by a yellow halo. Vision can vary widely, from unaffected to no perception of light. This condition doesn't get worse, but it can be associated with pituitary abnormalities, including poor growth and diabetes insipidus.

- **Megalopapilla.** In this very rare condition, the optic disk appears normal but is much larger than a standard disk. It generally doesn't affect optic nerve function.

- **Optic disk pit.** This refers to an oval or round depression in the optic disk. Usually, this affects only one eye. Children with an optic disk pit may feel like they have a blind spot. Vision sharpness isn't typically affected. Macular detachments are common with this condition and usually cause central vision loss later in life.

- **Optic disk drusen.** These are small dots that appear in the nerve or disk and gradually calcify. They're not typically visible with the naked eye early in a child's life. Eventually, they become visible as calcification progresses and the nerve fibers waste away. Many children with optic disk drusen have problems with peripheral vision later in life.

Acquired

Acquired diseases due to injury may cause cupping, swelling and wasting.

- **Cupping.** Cupping describes an increase in the middle depression of the optic nerve head. Conditions that produce increases in eye pressure, such as glaucoma, are common causes.

- **Optic neuritis.** This inflammation of the optic nerve causes the nerve to swell. Optic neuritis is thought to be an autoimmune disorder, which causes the body to attack its optic nerve tissue. Optic neuritis symptoms include a sudden and significant loss of vision in both eyes, headaches, painful eye movement, and decreased perception of color, brightness and peripheral vision. Possible triggers include a recent fever, viral illness and optic nerve infections. Treatment may not always be necessary, as vision may correct itself spontaneously. Recovery can take weeks to months. Intravenous (IV) corticosteroids may help speed up the healing process. A small number of children don't recover their vision.

Retinopathy of prematurity

Retinopathy of prematurity is an eye disorder caused by abnormal blood vessel growth in the retina of premature infants — generally those children born before week 31 of pregnancy and weighing 2.75 pounds or less at birth.

In retinopathy of prematurity, blood vessels swell and overgrow in the light-sensitive layer of nerves in the retina located at the back of the eye. When the condition is advanced, the abnormal retinal vessels extend into the jellylike substance (vitreous) that fills the eye's center. These vessels may scar the retina and stress its attachment to the back of the eye, causing partial or complete retinal detachment and potential blindness.

Treatment for retinopathy of prematurity depends on the severity of the condition. In most cases, retinopathy of prematurity resolves without treatment, causing no damage. Advanced retinopathy of prematurity, however, can lead to permanent vision problems or blindness. Some of the treatments have their own side effects.

Newer research has shown promise in treating advanced cases of retinopathy of prematurity with a combination of treatments:

- **Laser therapy.** It is the standard treatment for advanced retinopathy of prematurity. Laser therapy burns away the area around the retina's edge, which doesn't contain normal blood vessels but may contain abnormal ones. This procedure typically saves sight in the central part of the visual field but at the cost of side (peripheral) vision.

- **Cryotherapy.** This procedure, rarely performed in the United States, uses an instrument to freeze a specific part of the eye that extends beyond the retina's edges. Outcomes from laser therapy are generally better. Similar to laser therapy, the treatment destroys some peripheral vision.

- **Medications.** Drugs, including anti-vascular endothelial growth factor (anti-VEGF) drugs, are being researched as treatment options. Anti-VEGF drugs work by blocking the overgrowth of blood vessels in the retina. The medication is injected into the eye.

Although no drugs have received Food and Drug Administration approval specifically to treat retinopathy of prematurity, some medications approved

for other uses, such as bevacizumab (Avastin), are being explored as alternatives or additional therapies. Studies have shown that anti-VEGF drugs may improve outcomes when used in conjunction with laser therapy, but more research is needed to ensure effectiveness and safety.

Inherited retinal diseases

Many disorders that appear in childhood can affect the light-sensing tissue at the back of the eye, known as the retina. A thorough eye exam by an ophthalmologist can help determine which condition may be affecting a child's eyesight.

Retinitis pigmentosa

Retinitis pigmentosa is the name for a group of hereditary disorders that affect the retina and lead to gradual vision loss. The condition may be a dominant, recessive or X-chromosome-linked trait.

Usually, retinitis pigmentosa first impacts night vision and peripheral vision. A child may have problems seeing things out the sides of the eyes or in dark or dimly lit places. As the vision loss progresses, it typically affects central vision, too.

How quickly vision loss occurs varies by the type of inherited retinitis pigmentosa. Some children lose sight early in life, while others have good vision well into middle age. In some cases, retinitis pigmentosa may be part of a larger syndrome that produces multiple symptoms, such as Usher syndrome, a rare inherited disorder that causes deafness and gradual vision loss. Cataracts may also develop with this syndrome.

Glasses that correct refractive errors, removal of cataracts, and treatment of retina swelling with medication can help vision. Some research has suggested that supplementation with vitamin A may slow vision loss, but this is controversial. Research into potential treatments such as gene therapy, stem cell therapy and artificial retinas is ongoing.

Stargardt disease

Stargardt disease is a disorder that causes damage to the macula of the eye, which is located in the center of the retina. The macula is responsible for clear, forward-looking vision. The disorder damages parts of the retina called cones and rods, which help detect light, visual details and color. You may also see this condition referred to as Stargardt macular degeneration or juvenile macular degeneration.

A recessive gene mutation most commonly causes Stargardt. It usually triggers vision loss during childhood or adolescence, though vision problems can also begin in adulthood. How fast vision loss occurs varies by child. For children with earlier vision loss, Stargardt disease tends to progress rapidly. For others, it may be more gradual.

While people with Stargardt generally don't become blind, vision loss can progress to 20/200 or worse. A child with the disorder may see gray, black or hazy spots in his or her central vision or notice the eyes don't adjust when going from light to dark environments. Bright light may cause increased sensitivity. Some children develop color blindness or lose some peripheral vision as they age.

There's no treatment for Stargardt disease, so the focus is on preventing vision loss from worsening and providing coping strategies. Research continues into treatments such as medications to reduce retinal damage, gene therapy and stem cell-based therapies.

Leber congenital amaurosis

Leber congenital amaurosis is the name for a group of inherited conditions that typically appear by the time a child is 6 months old. It is the most common cause of inherited blindness in children and occurs because of a problem in the eyes' light-detecting portions. Leber congenital amaurosis is a recessive genetic mutation.

The first symptom is often uncontrolled eye movement (nystagmus, described earlier in this chapter), which typically occurs in the first few months of life. As time goes on, the child may experience poor vision, difficulties following objects with the eyes, light sensitivity, slow pupil response and increased touching of the eyes. Other problems also may develop, including cataracts and glaucoma.

Vision is usually 20/200 or worse and may seem to improve for a short time, then eventually decline. Certain genetic mutations that cause Leber congenital amaurosis also may make a child more likely to have kidney failure.

Gene therapy called voretigene neparvovec-rzyl (Luxturna) has recently been approved to treat specific forms of Leber congenital amaurosis caused by a mutation in the RPE65 gene. How long the benefits last or how the therapy affects disease progression isn't known. Glasses to correct vision problems and low-vision aids also can help children cope with the condition.

Cone-rod dystrophy

Cone-rod dystrophy is the name for a large group of inherited retinal diseases that damage the retina's light-sensing cones and rods, leading to severe vision loss. As the cones and rods deteriorate, sharp vision and extreme sensitivity to light may occur. These symptoms typically emerge in childhood.

Eventually, blind spots in the central field of vision, color blindness and loss of peripheral vision occur, leading to legal blindness by adulthood. Recessive, dominant and X-chromosome genetic mutations cause this condition.

There's no treatment for cone-rod dystrophy. Measures such as avoiding bright lights and using visual aids may help slow the disease's progression. Researchers are studying potential treatments, including gene therapy, stem cell therapy and retinal implants.

Retinoblastoma

Retinoblastoma is the most common form of cancer to affect the eye of a child. It occurs when nerve cells in the retina develop genetic mutations. These mutations cause the cells to continue growing and multiplying rather than dying as healthy cells do. The accumulating mass of cells forms a tumor.

In most cases, it's not clear what causes the genetic mutations that lead to retinoblastoma. However, children can inherit a genetic mutation from their parents. Inherited retinoblastoma tends to occur at an early age and in both eyes.

Signs and symptoms associated with retinoblastoma are uncommon. Sometimes a white color in the center circle of the eye (pupil) is visible when shining a light into the eye — such as when taking a flash photograph. Other possible signs and symptoms include eyes that appear to be looking in different directions, eye redness and eye swelling. Diagnosing retinoblastoma early, when the tumor is small, is the best chance at preserving vision and saving the child's life.

Treatment of pediatric retinoblastoma depends on the size and location of the tumor, whether the cancer has spread to areas other than the eye, and a child's overall health. The goal of treatment is to cure the cancer and, if possible, preserve vision.

Treatment includes:

- **Chemotherapy.** Medication is used to kill cancer cells. It may be administered in pill form or given through a blood vessel. Newer chemotherapy delivers drugs directly to the tumor through a tiny tube (catheter) in an artery in the eye or via an injection. In children with retinoblastoma, chemotherapy may help shrink a tumor so that another treatment, such as radiation therapy, cryotherapy or laser therapy, may be used to treat the remaining cancer cells. This may improve the chances that a child won't need surgery.

- **Radiation therapy.** Treatment may be delivered via internal radiation (brachytherapy), which involves placing a small disk of radioactive material into the eye with the goal of slowly destroying the tumor. External beam radiation delivers high-energy beams to the tumor from a large machine outside of the body. Because of side effects, it's typically reserved for children with advanced retinoblastoma and those for whom other treatments haven't worked.
- **Laser therapy (laser photocoagulation).** A laser is used to destroy blood vessels that supply oxygen and nutrients to the tumor.

- **Cold treatments (cryotherapy).** This procedure uses a repeated process of freezing and thawing to kill cancer cells. A very cold substance, such as liquid nitrogen, is placed in or near the cancer cells. Once the cells freeze, the cold substance is removed, and the cells thaw.
- **Surgery.** Removal of the eye may help prevent the spread of cancer to other parts of the body. An eye implant is typically placed immediately following the eyeball removal. Muscles that control eye movement are attached to the implant. After healing, a custom-made artificial eye that matches the child's healthy eye may be placed over the implant. The artificial eye will not restore vision.

Retinoblastoma cells can invade further into the eye and nearby structures. Retinoblastoma can also spread (metastasize) to other areas of the body, including the brain and spine. Additionally, children with the inherited form of retinoblastoma have an increased risk of developing different types of cancers in any part of the body in the years after treatment. For this reason, children with inherited retinoblastoma should have regular exams to screen for other cancers.

With most childhood eye diseases, the best way to improve or preserve vision is to find and treat the condition early. Vision screenings in children should begin at birth and occur regularly throughout childhood. For more information on screenings, see Chapter 9.

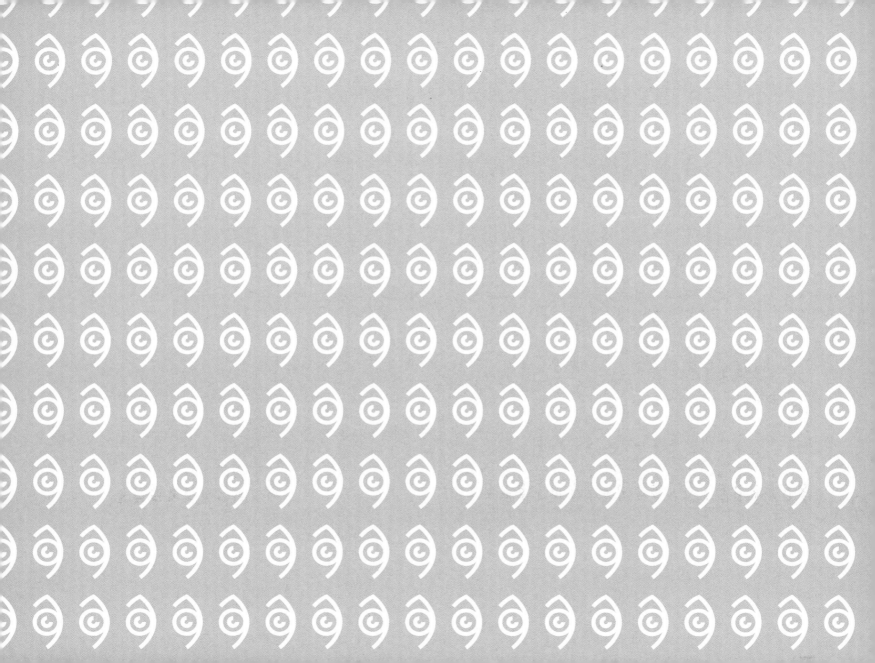

9

Protecting your vision

Is poor vision inevitable as you grow older? Not necessarily. Everyone's vision changes with age, but there are steps that you can take to protect your sight and reduce your risk of some eye diseases.

In fact, there are many things you can do to prevent eye injuries and vision problems. They include getting regular eye exams and controlling chronic medical conditions that can affect vision, such as diabetes and high blood pressure.

Preventive steps also include wearing protective eyewear in situations that may endanger your eyes and developing good work habits to avoid eyestrain. Even what you eat may make a difference.

In this chapter, you'll learn about healthy habits that can help optimize your eyesight today and nurture your vision for years to come. As you read the chapter, consider how your current habits compare with the recommended steps for protecting your eyesight.

Congratulate yourself on those measures you're already taking. Also identify areas for improvement, and set a goal for making positive changes. It can be difficult to alter your lifestyle habits, but protecting your sight is an excellent motivator to do so.

GET REGULAR EYE EXAMS

It likely comes as no surprise that eye exams are key. Routine eye exams are one of the best ways to protect your vision. A complete eye exam includes a series of

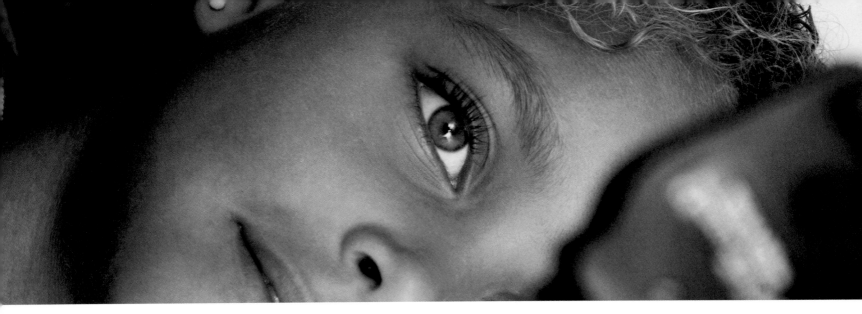

tests that evaluate different aspects of visual physiology and eye health.

Your eye doctor may examine your eyes' exterior and ask you to look at various objects through an array of lenses. Dilating eye drops may be applied that cause the openings at the front of your eyes (pupils) to widen. This allows the doctor, with the assistance of a bright light, to examine the inside of your eyeball and get a good view of the retina.

All of these tests provide important information about your visual acuity, depth perception, color vision, eye muscle movement, peripheral vision, eye pressure and the manner in which your pupils respond to light. The tests help detect eye problems in their early stages — when they're usually the most treatable.

Regularly scheduled eye exams also allow your eye doctor to:

- Adjust prescription changes to your vision brought on by aging
- Diagnose eye disease
- Identify and reduce sources of eye-strain and fatigue
- Provide tips on taking care of your eyes
- Make sure your vision is as good as it needs to be

If you wait for symptoms to develop before seeing an eye doctor, you may have waited too long. That's because many eye disorders, including macular degeneration, glaucoma and diabetic retinopathy, can do serious, irreparable damage to your vision before you experience symptoms.

Eye exam schedules

Several factors determine how frequently you need an eye exam. These factors include your age, your overall health and your risk of developing eye disease. Follow these general guidelines from the American Academy of Ophthalmology.

Young children

Among infants and toddlers, eye exams are important for detecting vision problems and risk factors that could threaten the healthy growth and development of a child's eyes.

You can usually count on your child's pediatrician or primary care provider to include eye exams for your child. However, if you have a family history of childhood eye problems, you may want to consult an eye specialist.

Screening for common childhood eye conditions, such as crossed eyes (strabismus), lazy eye (amblyopia) and drooping eyelid (ptosis), is typically part of a child's eye checkup. Once your child is about 3 years old, he or she will be ready for vision testing to detect refractive errors, such as nearsightedness, farsightedness and astigmatism.

In general, young children should have eye exams:

- At birth
- Between 6 months and 1 year old
- Between 1 and 3 years old
- Between 3 and 5 years old
- At age 5 and older

School-age children

After age 5, eye exams are recommended every 1 to 2 years if your child has no symptoms of eye disease and there's no family history of childhood vision problems.

Your child may need more-frequent eye exams and monitoring if you have a family history of childhood vision problems or your child has a condition that's known to put the eyes at risk, such as diabetes or thyroid disease.

Your child's pediatrician or primary care provider may continue to provide eye exams for your child at this age. Your child may be referred to an eye specialist if a structural or vision problem is detected during a routine exam.

Adults

In general, if you're healthy and you aren't exhibiting any symptoms of eye disease, the American Academy of Ophthalmology recommends that you have your vision checked at the following intervals:

- Every 5 to 10 years in your 20s and 30s
- Every 2 to 4 years between ages 40 and 54
- Every 1 to 3 years between ages 55 and 64
- Every 1 to 2 years at age 65 and beyond

You may need to have your eyes checked more frequently if you:

- Wear glasses or contact lenses
- Have a family history of eye disease
- Had an eye injury

- Have a chronic disease that puts you at greater risk of eye disease, such as diabetes

If you don't like the idea of wearing glasses or contact lenses, don't let that deter you from scheduling an appointment. An eye examination is the best way for your vision to be assessed and the risks to your eye health identified. Then you can develop an action plan for minimizing those risks and improving your vision, if needed.

Your action plan may involve the use of eyeglasses or contact lenses, but not always. If you have mild vision problems and your uncorrected vision isn't bothering you — you can still pass a driver's test and safely perform regular day-to-day activities — then you may not need to use corrective lenses. Going without corrective lenses won't make your vision any worse.

Who gives eye exams?

Eye examinations and routine eye care may involve the skills of three different professionals — ophthalmologists, optometrists and opticians.

BE PREPARED FOR YOUR EYE APPOINTMENT

During an exam, your eye doctor will likely ask questions about your personal and family medical history, in addition to examining your eyes and performing a variety of tests. Be prepared to answer the following questions as honestly and completely as possible, particularly if it's been several years since your previous visit. Take medical records to your eye appointment, if necessary.

- What vision problems are you currently having? What problems have you had in the past?
- If you wear eyeglasses or contact lenses, are you happy with them? If not, what is bothering you?
- Have you ever been diagnosed with a chronic disease or other health condition? If so, which ones?
- Are you currently taking any medications?
- Do you have any allergies?
- Do you have a family history of eye disease, such as macular degeneration, cataracts or glaucoma?
- Do you have a family history of chronic disease that affects vision, such as diabetes, high blood pressure or heart disease?

All of this information can help your eye doctor assess your risk of eye disease and evaluate your eye health.

Ophthalmologists

Ophthalmologists are medical doctors who specialize in eye problems. They're licensed to practice medicine and surgery. Ophthalmologists undergo at least four years of training beyond medical school focused on eye anatomy, physiology and disease. Some ophthalmologists choose to specialize in a specific area, such as glaucoma treatment and care. This requires additional training.

Ophthalmologists can provide eye exams and prescribe and fit corrective lenses. They can diagnose and treat complex eye disorders and perform corrective surgeries. Some ophthalmologists may limit the range of their services to treat specific eye diseases or perform a specific type of surgery.

Optometrists

Optometrists attend optometry school after college and receive a doctor of optometry (O.D.) degree upon completion. They're trained and licensed to provide many eye care services, such as evaluating your vision, prescribing corrective lenses, diagnosing common eye disorders and treating certain eye diseases with medications. For complex eye problems or for conditions requiring surgery, your optometrist may refer you to an ophthalmologist.

Opticians

Opticians are technicians who are trained to fill prescriptions for eyeglasses and contact lenses. They don't test vision or write prescriptions but can dispense medications requested by optometrists and ophthalmologists.

Ophthalmologists, optometrists and opticians often work together to provide the best possible eye care. Consider the qualifications, experience and services provided when selecting an individual or group practice for your eye care.

SIGNS OF AN EYE EMERGENCY

Recognizing the warning signs of an eye emergency and seeking immediate attention are critical to maintaining healthy vision. If you notice any of these signs and symptoms, schedule an appointment with your eye doctor as soon as possible, even if you've recently had an eye exam:

- Sudden onset of hazy or blurred vision
- Eye pain
- Flashes of light, dark spots or ghostlike images in your visual field
- Halos or rainbows that form around lights
- Lines and edges

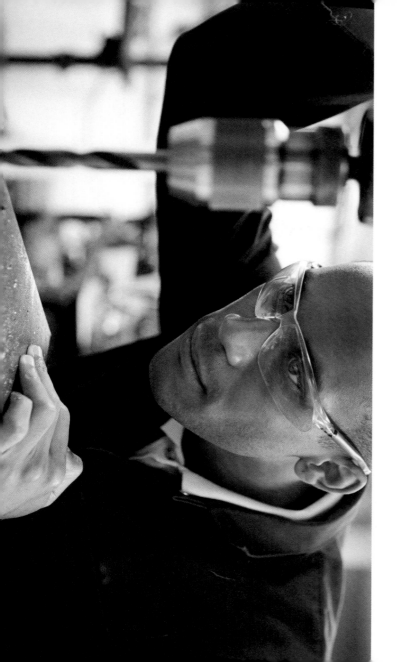

USE PROTECTIVE EYEWEAR

One of the most effective ways to protect your vision is to wear safety glasses or goggles in situations that could potentially injure your eyes. According to the National Society to Prevent Blindness, studies show that proper eye protection could have prevented nearly 90% of all impact injuries to the eye.

At work

Chemical splashes, pesticide fumes, flying particles of metal, glass and wood — these are among the workplace hazards that put your eyes at risk. If you work in an agricultural or industrial setting or in a chemical laboratory, there is a very real possibility of sustaining a serious eye injury.

Know the eye hazards at your job and always wear appropriate protective eyewear. Also, be sure to eliminate hazards by being properly trained to use chemical fume hoods, machine guards, work screens or other engineering controls.

If your job carries a risk of eye injury, your employer is required by law to provide you with safety glasses. The type of protective eyewear you need depends on your job. Make sure you have the right gear for the work you're doing — whether it's safety glasses with side shields, goggles, a face shield or a helmet. Then wear it faithfully.

At home

Today, nearly half of all eye injuries occur at home, and that number continues to rise. Eye injuries can occur while mowing the lawn, clipping hedges and bushes, and using all manner of power tools. They can occur while working with cleaning solvents and lawn chemicals, preparing foods that splatter grease or oil, or opening champagne bottles.

Be sure to keep all of your tools in good condition and use other safety precautions, such as placing grease shields on frying pans.

Many common household products can be extremely harmful if they come in

HOW TO HANDLE AN EYE INJURY

Immediately see an eye specialist or go to a hospital emergency room, even if an eye injury seems minor. The full extent of the damage isn't always apparent.

If you sustain a blunt injury or cut to your eye:

- Don't rub your eye (which can cause more tissue damage) or rinse your eye.
- Don't put any ointment or medication on your eye.
- Don't try to remove an object stuck in your eye.
- Gently cover the eye with some type of shield and seek medical attention. For example, tape the bottom of a foam cup against your eye socket.
- Avoid taking acetaminophen (Tylenol, others), ibuprofen (Advil, Motrin IB, others), naproxen sodium (Aleve) or aspirin. These medications may increase bleeding.

If you get a chemical in your eye:

- Immediately flush the eye with lukewarm tap water to remove any chemical residue. Try to pull the eyelids open as wide as possible and flood the eye with a steady stream of water for 15 to 20 minutes. Tilt your head toward the injured side so that the chemical does not wash into the uninjured eye.
- After rinsing the eye, cover it with a soft pad.
- Seek emergency medical care. Take the chemical container with you, or write the product name on a slip of paper and take that.

If you have a foreign object or particle in your eye:

- Don't rub your eye.
- If it's a minor issue, such as a small particle of dust, try blinking several times and allow tears to remove the particle.
- If blinking doesn't work, try to flush out the object. Fill a small glass with lukewarm water or saline solution. Rest the rim of the glass against your eye socket and pour the fluid into your eye, keeping your eye open.
- Don't try to remove an object that's embedded in the eyeball or that makes closing your eye difficult.

contact with your eyes. These products include detergents, drain cleaners, disinfectants, solvents, oven cleaners, and any products containing bleach, ammonia, chlorine, alkali and lye. Follow the instructions and always fall on the side of caution. Remember to never mix cleaning agents together.

It's a good idea to wear protective eyewear when doing home repairs, certain hobbies and activities that pose a risk to your vision. Whether you're repairing the car, painting the house or cleaning the garage, wear safety goggles to keep dirt, rust, paint chips and other small particles from landing in your eyes. If a child is helping you, make sure that he or she wears protective eyewear as well.

At play

A ball thrown at high speed can cause serious damage to your eye. Unintentional finger pokes during a recreational game may scrape or tear your cornea. Eye trauma may result from trips and falls. In fact, tens of thousands of sports- and recreation-related eye injuries occur every year.

Eye injuries are common in baseball, basketball and racket sports. Boxing and

SUN SMARTS

Besides wearing sunglasses when you're outdoors, follow these tips to keep your eyes protected from the sun:

- Wear a wide-brimmed hat or cap. A large amount of sunlight comes from directly overhead and can slip past most sunglasses.
- Never look at the sun directly, even through sunglasses. Doing so can permanently damage your eyes. You can also hurt your eyes by routinely staring at the sun reflected on water.
- Wear protective sunscreen on your face and around your eyes, including on your eyelids.
- Avoid commercial tanning booths. If you do use them, make sure the salon gives you special protective goggles to wear.
- Many common medications — including antibiotics, antidepressants, diuretics, statins and nonsteroidal anti-inflammatory drugs (NSAIDs) — make your eyes more sensitive to light. Make sure you know if your medications are sun-sensitizing. If so, be extra cautious when outside. Wear sunglasses and a hat each time you go outside.
- If you have an eye disease, such as macular degeneration, you're at greater risk of UV-related eye damage. Protect your eyes whenever you go outside, no matter how briefly.

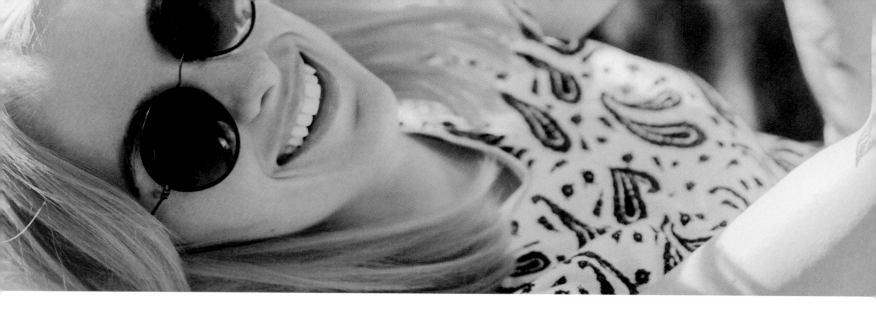

martial arts also pose a high risk of serious eye injuries.

Many injuries could be prevented with appropriate eyewear. Proper protection varies by activity. For basketball, racket sports and field hockey, impact-resistant eyewear made of polycarbonate plastic is a good bet. For baseball, ice hockey and lacrosse, consider a helmet with a strong, shatterproof, lightweight plastic face mask or wire shield. For the swimming pool, use goggles to block the eye-irritating effects of chemicals, such as chlorine.

Hard workouts may cause protective eyewear to fog up. If this happens, don't remove your eyewear during play for any reason. Wait until there's a break in the action or you have a chance to leave the game.

WEAR SUNGLASSES

Ultraviolet (UV) rays from the sun can damage your eyes as well as your skin. Long-term exposure to UV radiation can increase your risk of eye disease, particularly cataracts and age-related macular degeneration. Even artificial light sources, such as welding arcs or tanning lamps, are capable of burning the cornea and conjunctiva of your eye.

The best way to protect your eyes from the sun is to wear sunglasses designed to block UV radiation and eliminate glare. Sunglasses don't have to be expensive to be effective. Look for a pair of sunglasses that block 99% to 100% ultraviolet A and ultraviolet B light. To be even more

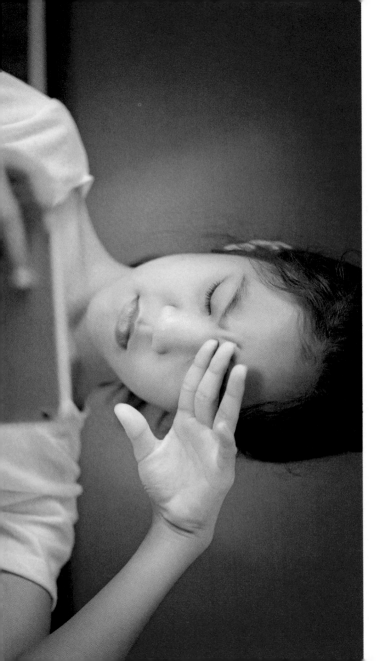

effective, they should fit close to your face or have wraparound frames.

Wear sunglasses anytime you're outdoors for more than a few minutes, including cloudy days. Even when clouds are blocking the sun, they don't block all UV radiation.

You can reduce glare — the light that bounces off smooth surfaces such as pavement, water, sand and snow — by choosing darker lenses that screen out visible light. Polarized lenses also reduce reflected glare. But polarization doesn't block UV radiation, so if you're buying polarizing lenses, check the label to make sure that they also provide maximum UV protection.

AVOID EYESTRAIN

Any type of work or activity that depends on intensive use of your eyes — such as driving, reading, doing crafts, or staring at a computer, smartphone or tablet — may cause eyestrain. This doesn't lead to permanent eye damage, but it can affect everyday vision.

Common signs and symptoms of eyestrain include:

- Eye fatigue
- Dry, itchy, watery or burning eyes
- Blurry or double vision
- Headaches
- Neck or back pain
- Increased sensitivity to light
- Squinting

Shed light on the subject

When doing intensive, close-up work, make sure that you have light that's well directed on what you're doing. And don't be shy about increasing the electrical power, if needed.

Although a standard-watt light bulb may be sufficient for a person with normal vision, a bulb with much higher wattage may be necessary if you have impaired vision. Whenever you change a bulb, make sure the light fixture can handle the wattage of the new bulb.

When reading

Try to position the light source behind you and direct the light onto the page. The light should be bright but not glaring. If you're reading at a desk, use a shaded light positioned in front of you. The shade will keep light from shining into your eyes.

When watching television

Keep the room softly illuminated while watching TV. Too much contrast between a screen and its dark surroundings can result in eyestrain.

When on devices

If you spend most of your day staring at a computer monitor, laptop, tablet or smartphone you're probably experiencing some eyestrain. For example, you may see color fringes or afterimages as you glance away from the screen.

Researchers don't believe this activity will have long-term consequences, but the symptoms can be unpleasant and disruptive.

Try these strategies to prevent eyestrain:
• **Take blinking breaks.** Many people blink less than normal while using a computer or other digital device. This can result in dry, irritated eyes. Make a conscious effort to blink more often. Blinking produces tears that help moisten and lubricate your eyes. Consider putting a note on your screen to remind you to blink.

• **Look away.** Intermittently force your eyes to focus on something other than your screen. Try following the 20-20-20 rule: Every 20 minutes, take your eyes off your computer or tablet and look at something 20 feet away for at least 20 seconds.

• **Change the pace.** Stand up and move around at least once every hour or so. Don't use a break from your computer monitor to respond to texts on your smartphone. Do something that doesn't involve a screen, such as taking a short walk for a water break. A few times a day, lean back and close your eyes for a few moments.

• **Pay attention to position.** Position screens directly in front of you, about 20 to 40 inches away from the tip of your nose. The center of the screen should be just below eye level so that you look down slightly. When you're using a desktop computer, place the keyboard directly in front of the monitor. If the keyboard is at an angle or to the side, your eyes may tire from having to constantly shift their focus.

• **Reduce glare.** Pay attention to the placement of your computer screen. The worst problems with glare are generally from light sources located above or behind you, including fluorescent lighting and sunlight. Also avoid placing the screen directly in front of a window or white wall. Consider a glare-reducing screen or anti-glare cover. And be sure to adjust your screen brightness so it's about the same as your surroundings. Keep lighting about half that of normal room lighting.

- **Keep screens clean.** Dust off your electronic devices regularly. Dust cuts down on contrast and may intensify the glare on your screens.
- **Get proper eyewear.** If you wear glasses or contact lenses, make sure the correction is right for computer work. Many lenses are intended for close-up reading and may not be optimal for long hours spent looking at a computer screen. Check into computer glasses. They allow you to focus your eyes on a computer screen, which is farther away than the distance at which reading material is normally held.

READ LABELS CAREFULLY

Some over-the-counter eye drops contain additives, or chemical preservatives that discourage bacteria growth once the bottle has been opened. These additives and preservatives can irritate your eyes or cause an allergic reaction. If your eyes or eyelids become more red, itchy or swollen after you apply the eye drops, stop using them and talk to your eye doctor.

Also, be sure to read — and follow — the recommended dosage for whatever eye drops you use. Administering some drops more frequently than recommended can cause problems. For example, if you use decongestive eye drops too often, a rebound effect may occur — the redness and irritation in the eye increases as the drops wear off.

If you're at risk of angle-closure glaucoma, don't use eye drops that contain antihistamines. They can provoke a glaucoma attack, causing nausea, vomiting, eye pain and the sudden onset of visual disturbances.

USE EYE DROPS PROPERLY

Over-the-counter eye drops can help prevent and relieve dry, irritated eyes. Eye drops can also soothe mild eye discomfort from allergies or other causes. Three types of eye drops are available without a prescription:

Lubricating eye drops

Lubricating eye drops, or artificial tears, help retain moisture and prevent it from evaporating, much as your own tears do. One or two drops of artificial tears can soothe irritated eyes, providing lubrication and comfort. If you choose a brand that doesn't contain preservatives, you can use them as often as needed. They're a good choice for computer eyestrain.

Decongestive eye drops

Decongestive eye drops, or vasoconstrictors, relieve redness by shrinking tiny blood vessels in the conjunctiva. One or two drops are effective for several hours and often soothe irritation. Improvement in eye symptoms should be prompt. If not, check with an eye doctor to see if this signals a more serious concern.

Allergy eye drops

Some eye drops include an antihistamine that provides relief from seasonal allergies such as hay fever. Use allergy eye drops no more than two or three times a day, or as instructed by your doctor.

How to use eye drops

To properly administer eye drops:

1. Tilt your head back and gently pull your lower lid away from the eye to form a small pocket. Let the drop fall into the pocket. Don't allow the tip of the bottle to brush against the surface of your eye or your eyelid.

2. Close your eye gently and don't blink. Don't squeeze the lids shut, which may force fluid out of the eye.

3. Use your index finger to apply gentle pressure at the inside corner of your closed eye. This prevents the drop from draining immediately through the tear duct.

4. Keep your eye closed for a minute. Wipe any excess drops and tears from your lids with a tissue. Then open your eye.

QUIT SMOKING

Cigarette smoke harms nearly every organ of your body — your eyes are no exception. Smoke, like any air pollutant, can irritate and redden eyes. What's more, smoking is a risk factor for cataracts, macular degeneration, diabetic retinopathy, ischemic optic neuropathy and retinal vascular occlusions.

If you smoke, you have another powerful reason to quit — the opportunity to protect your eyesight. There are many resources available to help you quit smoking. You can find the knowledge, tools and support from your health care provider or trusted online organizations and local groups within your own community.

EAT FOR EYE HEALTH

You've probably heard that carrots are good for your eyes. But what about the benefits of other foods?

Is there a healthy diet that protects your vision? The answer is maybe. Scientists believe a lack of certain nutrients, including some vitamins, carotenoids and fats, may be one of the reasons why your macula and other parts of the eye may start to deteriorate with age. Upping your intake of these nutrients may help protect your eyes from age-related macular degeneration and other eye diseases.

Eating for eye health doesn't require you to add uncommon or unappetizing foods to your daily diet. An eye-friendly diet is a healthy, balanced diet that also protects you from other serious diseases such as heart disease and diabetes, and helps you maintain a healthy weight.

Fruits and vegetables

Carotenoids are a family of nutrients found in richly colored fruits and vegetables. Your body converts some carotenoids into vitamins; for example, turning beta carotene into vitamin A. Carotenoid nutrients are highly concentrated in the eye's retina and often become significantly reduced when the macula starts to deteriorate.

Many carotenoids have antioxidant properties. Your body — and your eyes — use the antioxidants to combat unstable molecules in the bloodstream, called free radicals. Free radicals perform a number of useful functions in the body, but a surplus can damage normal cells in a process called oxidation. Oxidation is thought to play a role in the development of eye diseases such as macular degeneration, glaucoma and cataracts.

Lutein and zeaxanthin

Accumulating evidence indicates that lutein and zeaxanthin may play important

SOURCES OF ANTIOXIDANTS

A wide variety of fresh foods can provide you with the antioxidants you need for good eye health.

Vitamin E. Good sources of vitamin E include vegetable oils and a variety of products made from them. Wheat germ, nuts and avocados also contain relatively high amounts of vitamin E.

Vitamin C. Good sources of vitamin C include green and red bell peppers, collard greens, broccoli, spinach, tomatoes, potatoes, strawberries and other berries, oranges, grapefruit, and other citrus fruits.

Carotenoids. Good sources of carotenoids include deep yellow, dark green and red vegetables and fruits, including carrots, winter squash, sweet potatoes, broccoli, bell peppers, tomatoes, papayas, cantaloupe, mangoes, apricots and watermelon. Beta carotene is the best-known carotenoid but not the only one. Lutein and zeaxanthin are found in dark green leafy vegetables, including spinach, kale, collard greens, mustard greens, Swiss chard, watercress and parsley. Red bell peppers and romaine lettuce contain smaller amounts of these two carotenoids.

roles in preventing and reducing cataracts and age-related macular degeneration. These two carotenoids, which are highly concentrated in the macula, seem to filter out damaging radiation from sunlight. Both are also strong antioxidants, protecting your eyes against oxidation.

Lutein and zeaxanthin are found at high levels in dark green leafy vegetables and herbs. That includes foods such as spinach, kale, collard greens, mustard greens, Swiss chard, watercress and parsley. Lutein and zeaxanthin also are present in orange bell peppers and egg yolks.

SOME SUCCESS WITH SUPPLEMENTS

Several years ago, results from a study called the Age-Related Eye Disease Study (AREDS) provided encouraging news regarding vision and diet. The study, funded by the National Eye Institute, included people with dry macular degeneration, at different stages of the disease. Some participants were given a daily high-dose vitamin and mineral supplement of vitamin A (beta carotene), vitamin C, vitamin E, zinc and copper. Others were given an inactive pill (placebo). Over a five-year period, the participants were closely monitored, and outcomes from the two groups were compared.

Individuals in the supplement group lowered their risk of advanced stages of age-related macular degeneration by about 25%. They also reduced their risk of vision loss due to macular degeneration by about 19%. However, only participants in the intermediate and advanced stages of macular degeneration benefited from the supplements. Participants with no age-related macular degeneration or in early stages of the disease saw no benefit.

A few years later, the same research group conducted a second study called AREDS2 to determine if they could improve the formulation. Based on this study, the AREDS2 formula was altered. Beta carotene was removed and lutein and zeaxanthin were added.

The AREDS and AREDS2 formulations are sold at local pharmacies. You might consider taking the formulations if you have intermediate dry macular degeneration in one or both eyes or advanced dry macular degeneration in one eye but not the other and you want to keep the disease from progressing to a more advanced stage. At this point, there's little evidence that the AREDS formulation can prevent macular degeneration, especially among those with a family history of the disease.

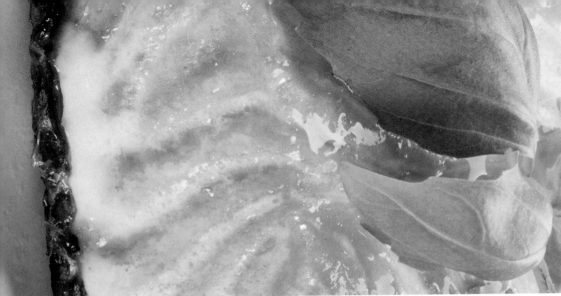
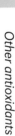
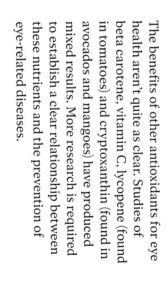

Other antioxidants

The benefits of other antioxidants for eye health aren't quite as clear. Studies of beta carotene, vitamin C, lycopene (found in tomatoes) and cryptoxanthin (found in avocados and mangoes) have produced mixed results. More research is required to establish a clear relationship between these nutrients and the prevention of eye-related diseases.

Though not all evidence is conclusive, including a wide variety of fruits and vegetables in your diet is an excellent way to promote good eye health. It's also good for your overall health in general. Try eating at least five servings of fruits and vegetables each day.

The wider the variety, the better. The most colorful fruits and vegetables — yellow, orange, red, blue and dark green — contain nutrients that are the most highly concentrated in your eyes. But this doesn't mean that they're the only ones you should eat. Most fresh produce is beneficial to your health.

Fish

A healthy retina contains a high concentration of omega-3 fatty acids. Studies show that a diet high in fish and omega-3 fatty acids may reduce the risk of advanced macular degeneration. You can find omega-3 fatty acids in certain varieties of fish, such as salmon, tuna, halibut and herring. Omega-3 fatty acids can also be found in lesser amounts in flaxseed, chia seeds, walnuts and canola oil.

Supplements and vitamins

If you eat a balanced diet, your eyes should be getting all of the nutrients they need. It's fine to take a daily vitamin and mineral supplement, but supplements aren't a substitute for a healthy diet.

Studies show that certain combinations of vitamins and minerals may slow the progress of an eye disorder (see page 175) but they don't appear to have any preventive effects. If you take daily supplements, don't exceed 100% of the Daily Value for each substance, unless your doctor advises otherwise.

Multivitamins

Observational studies indicate that multivitamins may lower the risk of cataracts, but these findings haven't been confirmed with clinical trials. It's possible the reduced risk may be due to other factors practiced by people taking the vitamins.

Zinc

One of the most common trace minerals in your body, zinc is concentrated in the retina. Although the role of zinc in eye health is unclear, some scientists speculate that a lack of zinc may contribute to macular degeneration.

A balanced diet usually provides you with adequate amounts of zinc, but researchers are studying the long-term effect of zinc supplements. There are dangers associated with high doses of zinc because it may reduce copper or iron absorption into your bloodstream. But it's possible that taking a zinc supplement may prevent macular degeneration from progressing to advanced stages.

THE LONG VIEW

Preserving your eyesight and reducing your risk of eye disease doesn't happen overnight. It may take years before you see positive results. In addition to benefits to your eyesight, adopting the healthy habits discussed in this chapter — such as eating more vegetables and fruits, quitting smoking, and reducing eyestrain — goes a long way toward improving your overall health and quality of life. So, what are you waiting for? Get started!

10

Correcting vision

If you need sharper vision, you're in good company. Approximately 180 million people in the U.S. — more than half of the population — use some form of corrective eyewear to help them see better. Good vision is essential for a variety of routine tasks that you perform every day, including driving, reading, walking, and operating tools and appliances.

Fortunately for most people, better vision is easy to attain. Eyeglasses and contact lenses are options for correcting the most common vision problems, such as nearsightedness, farsightedness and astigmatism. The difficulty of seeing objects up close (presbyopia), which comes with age, also can be effectively treated with eyeglasses. A wide variety of styles and options are available to suit your lifestyle and fashion sense.

If you'd rather not deal with eyeglasses or contact lenses, you may choose to have your vision corrected with refractive surgery. LASIK eye surgery is the most common form of refractive surgery, but other surgical options are available as well, depending on your vision needs.

Whatever you decide, a complete evaluation of your vision by an eye doctor is extremely important. Each person's eyes are different, and the best corrective measures are the ones that meet your specific needs. In deciding how to improve your eyesight, you and your eye doctor will also consider your personal preferences.

Understanding key differences among the various options will help you choose the correction that best suits your lifestyle.

COMMON VISION PROBLEMS

The intricate process of seeing, with so many complex interactions, can sometimes go wrong. The most common impairments to vision are usually caused by a focusing problem of the cornea or lens or by an abnormal shape of the eye. These problems can often be corrected with eyeglasses, contact lenses or surgery that adjusts the curvature of your cornea.

You see objects clearly when your cornea and lens focus light rays precisely on your retina (see illustrations below). If the focusing powers of your cornea and lens aren't matched perfectly to the length or shape of your eye, however, the point of sharpest focus will fall just short of or behind the retina. When that happens, the image you see is blurred.

COMMON VISION PROBLEMS

With normal vision (left), the arrow indicates that the point of focus falls on your retina, providing clear, sharp vision. With nearsightedness (center), the arrow indicates that the point of focus lies in front of your retina, making distant objects appear blurry. With farsightedness (right), the arrow indicates that the point of focus falls behind your retina, making close-up objects appear blurry.

Nearsightedness

If you're nearsighted — a condition called myopia — you see close objects clearly but objects farther away are blurry. Nearsightedness commonly occurs when your eye is slightly more elongated than normal. This causes light rays to be focused in front of instead of on the retina.

Even with an eye of normal length front to back, you can be nearsighted if your cornea or lens is too steeply curved, bending light rays into focus before they reach the retina.

Nearsightedness is often detected during childhood. Signs and symptoms of the condition include:

• Persistent squinting

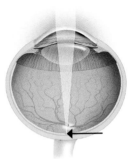
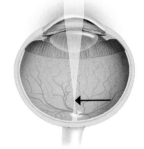
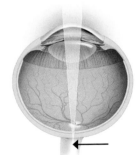

- Sitting very close to a television or movie screen
- Holding books very close to the face while reading
- Seeming unaware of objects or events taking place in the distance

Nearsightedness affects boys and girls equally and it tends to be hereditary. Early on, continued changes may require new corrective lenses more than once a year, but the condition tends to stabilize in the late teen years.

Farsightedness

When you're farsighted — a condition called hyperopia — you may see distant objects clearly but close objects are blurry. Very often, people are farsighted because their eyes are shorter than normal, so the sharpest point of focus falls behind the retina. Farsightedness may also stem from either a cornea or a lens that's flattened, weakening refractive power.

Farsightedness is usually present at birth and it tends to be hereditary. Most young people don't know they have the condition because their eyes' lenses are flexible and able to compensate for the condition. As they grow older, the lenses become less elastic and unable to make the necessary adjustments. In time, people who are farsighted will need corrective lenses for near vision, and some may eventually need correction for distance vision as well.

Signs and symptoms of farsightedness include:

- Nearby objects appearing blurry and needing to be held out to see them clearly
- Needing to squint to see clearly
- Eyestrain, including burning eyes, aching in and around the eyes, and — rarely — a headache
- General eye and brow discomfort after prolonged reading

Astigmatism

Astigmatism is a mild imperfection in the curvature of your cornea or lens that blurs vision at any distance. In a normal eye, the surface of the cornea or lens is curved equally and smoothly in all directions. That means when you're looking at a basketball, for example, the shape of the ball will appear as round or spherical.

Sometimes, a cornea or lens will have surface curvature in some directions that is different from surface curvature in other directions. That causes a vision problem. Light in the more sharply curved (steeper) directions is focused closer to the front of the eye. Light in the less curved (flatter) directions is focused farther from the front of the eye. The different points of sharp focus caused by the astigmatism create a blur in your vision.

In most cases, astigmatism is established in early childhood, but it may develop later after injury or disease. It frequently occurs in combination with nearsightedness or farsightedness. Astigmatism generally doesn't change throughout a

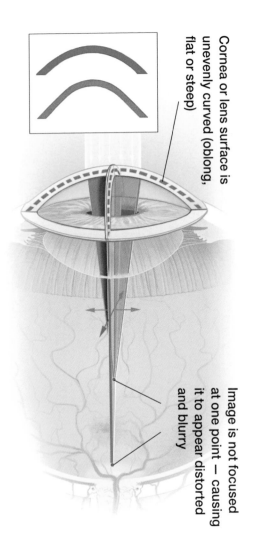

Cornea or lens surface is unevenly curved (oblong, flat or steep)

Image is not focused at one point — causing it to appear distorted and blurry

person's lifetime. Astigmatism is common and can be corrected with eyeglasses or contact lenses that counteract the problem. The lenses can correct near-sightedness or farsightedness at the same time. Another option is refractive surgery.

Presbyopia

The term *presbyopia* may not be familiar to you, but the condition is common. Presbyopia refers to your eyes' gradual loss of their ability to focus on nearby objects. It's a natural part of aging. About the time you're age 40 or older, you may notice that it's more difficult to read something at a customary distance from your eyes. You're forced to hold the text farther away, sometimes at arm's length, to see it clearly.

When you're young, the lenses in your eyes are very elastic, giving you a wide range of focus. They naturally thicken when you do close-up work to focus light directly on your retina. As you get older, the lenses gradually lose some of their elasticity, making it more difficult to focus on nearby objects. You may experience eyestrain and headaches from prolonged periods of reading or typing.

ASTIGMATISM AND VISION

Astigmatism is caused by the uneven curvature of your cornea or lens, which is unable to focus the light entering your eye at a single point. Instead, based on the differences in curvature, the light will be focused at multiple points, creating distorted, blurry vision.

You potentially can correct presbyopia with nonprescription reading glasses and contact lenses. The condition worsens with age, but by the time you're about age 65, your lenses have lost most of their elasticity and don't accommodate focal points anymore. At this time, changes to your prescription are less likely.

CORRECTIVE LENSES

Corrective lenses — whether they be eyeglasses, contact lenses or another type of lens — help resolve refractive errors caused by nearsightedness, farsightedness, astigmatism and presbyopia. Corrective lenses are custom-built to your vision needs and can be worn on or in front of your eyes to correct problems with the shape of your eye or the curvature of your cornea or lens.

It's helpful to think of corrective lenses as a group of prisms melded together. A scientific principle to know about prisms: Light passing through a prism is always

bent (refracted) toward the thickest part of the glass.

A concave lens, indicated by a minus sign on the first number (sphere) of your prescription, is thickest at the edges. It bends light outward. This kind of lens is used to correct nearsightedness by moving the point of focus a little farther to reach the retina. A convex lens, indicated by a plus sign, is thickest in the middle. It bends light inward. This kind of lens is used to correct farsightedness.

Your prescription from a routine eye exam includes a refractive power to correct your vision problem. The higher the prescription numbers, the stronger the prescription. The numbers also determine the shape and thickness of the lens. The more refraction required, the thicker the lens needs to be.

On your prescription, you may also have a number labeled "add." This indicates an additional power for your correction to help with near vision. Additional power is

POOR COLOR VISION

Most people who have what's commonly known as colorblindness aren't really colorblind. That would mean they see objects only in black and white. Actually, their problem is distinguishing between certain shades of color. Most people with poor color vision can't tell the difference between shades of red and green.

Poor color vision is usually inherited, although some eye diseases and certain medications also may cause it. The problem arises from chemical deficiencies in the cone cells. Defects can be mild, moderate or severe.

most often prescribed to individuals with presbyopia.

There may be two additional numbers on your prescription, defined as cylinder and axis. These numbers indicate the amount (cylinder) and direction (axis) of astigmatism. There are two different ways to write this number, either with a minus sign or a plus sign in front of the cylinder number. If you're given a prescription in one format, it may look very different, yet be the same as a prescription written in the other format. Be careful if you compare prescriptions and one has a minus sign and the other has a plus sign in front of the cylinder. An eye specialist will know how to make the conversion to either system, so it won't matter which version you have.

EYEGLASSES

Eyeglasses are available from many locations — small optical shops, department stores, discount centers, nationwide optical chains or online. When selecting a pair to meet your needs, there are a number of things to consider.

Lens material

Eyeglass lenses are made of plastic or glass, and for the most part, your vision can be corrected with either type of lens. The material you choose is often based on factors of safety and lifestyle. A majority of eyeglass wearers choose plastic lenses, which tend to be lighter than glass lenses, but glass also has advantages.

Plastic

Plastic lenses are lighter weight and more impact resistant than glass lenses. They're also easier to tint. Although they scratch more easily than do glass lenses, plastic lenses routinely come with a scratch-resistant coating. High-index plastic is a thin, lightweight option for moderate to strong prescriptions. Hard-resin plastic is a little thicker but considerably less expensive than the high-index kind. Polycarbonate is the strongest plastic available and a preferred choice for kids and use in safety glasses.

Glass

Glass lenses are more scratch resistant than are plastic lenses, but they can be almost twice as heavy. For many people, the weight of glass lenses is a drawback, especially with big frames. Glass also can break or chip. In the event that eyeglasses with glass lenses are hit while being worn, the glass could shatter and damage one or both eyes. In terms of eye protection, glass is a poor choice.

Lens coatings

Another consideration when purchasing eyeglasses is the coating placed on the lens material.

Scratch protection

A clear coating is often applied to plastic lenses to make them more scratch resistant. It's best that both sides of the lenses are treated because it's easy to scratch the inside surface of a lens while cleaning it. Scratch protection is often included in the cost but it may be an additional charge.

Anti-reflection coating

Reflection and glare are bothersome, particularly if you have a stronger prescription, which increases glare. Placing anti-reflection (AR) coating on your lenses reduces the light that's reflected off of them and improves vision. Anti-reflection coating also helps keep the lenses clear, allowing others to see your eyes better.

Ultraviolet protection

Ultraviolet (UV) rays may contribute to age-related eye diseases such as cataracts and macular degeneration. High-index and polycarbonate plastic lenses typically have UV protection included, so don't be talked into paying extra for UV protection you may have already purchased.

Anti-fog coating

An up-and-coming technology is anti-fog coating. You may be familiar with foggy eyeglasses when you walk into a warm house from the cold outdoors or when wearing a face mask. Researchers are looking to prevent this problem, but the

BASIC LENS SHAPES

A concave lens (left) corrects for nearsightedness. The dashed green line indicates how the corrective lens shifts the uncorrected point of focus back to the retina. A convex lens (right) corrects for farsightedness. The dashed green line indicates how the corrective lens moves the uncorrected point of focus forward to the retina. Convex lenses are commonly used in reading glasses.

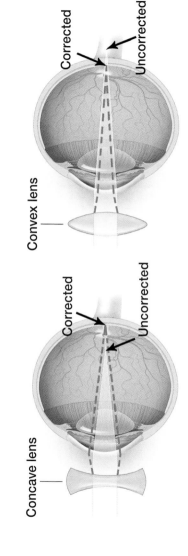

Concave lens
Corrected
Uncorrected

Convex lens
Corrected
Uncorrected

YOUR EYEGLASSES PRESCRIPTION

Certain conventions and terminology are used in a typical prescription for corrective lenses. If you don't know what the numbers mean, a prescription can seem quite confusing. Here's an example of the prescription for a person who is nearsighted and also has astigmatism.

	Sphere	Cylinder	Axis	
OD	-2.75	+2.25	90	
OS	-2.00	+1.75	90	+1.50 add

- OD (oculus dexter) is the right eye, sometimes listed as RE.
- OS (oculus sinister) is the left eye, sometimes listed as LE.
- Sphere is the correction measurement for your nearsightedness or farsightedness. A minus sign indicates a concave lens, which corrects nearsightedness. A plus sign indicates a convex lens, which corrects farsightedness.
- Cylinder is the correction measurement for astigmatism. This may be blank if you have no astigmatism or your astigmatism is so slight that it doesn't need to be corrected. Cylinder may have either a minus sign or a plus sign in front of it, depending on the format used by your eye specialist. When comparing two prescriptions, they may be the same, but look completely different if they have different signs in front of the cylinder.
- Axis shows the direction of the astigmatism correction in the lens — the direction in degrees from horizontal. It can be anywhere from 1 to 180 degrees, with 90 degrees being an up-and-down (vertical) line.
- +1.50 add at the bottom of the prescription indicates the need for additional power in the lens, in this case, an additional bifocal lens power will be needed for close-up work.

The numbers in the sphere and cylinder columns are units of lens power called diopters, which are based on how much bending (refraction) occurs when light passes through the lens. Diopters can increase or decrease in quarter (0.25) increments. The higher the numbers in the prescription, the more refraction needed to correct your vision, and the thicker your lens will be.

technology remains exploratory and still isn't widely available to the public.

Lens treatments

When purchasing eyeglasses, you also have the option of additional lens features that can help accommodate specific vision needs or your personal preferences.

Photochromic

Commonly called transition lenses, photochromic lenses are chemically treated to adjust to different levels of brightness. They get dark like sunglasses in direct sunlight and become clear in a dimly lit room. Photochromic lenses require UV light in order to darken or lighten, so they won't become darker while you're inside a vehicle (the windshield absorbs the UV light). Therefore, you may need to keep a pair of sunglasses in the car.

Tint

Unlike photochromic lenses, tinted lenses remain a constant shade in all levels of brightness. Adding color to your glasses can help if you're especially sensitive to light or you simply want to make a fashion statement. Almost any color can be selected for a tint. Sunglasses are often gray or brown. Some people feel that a yellow tint improves contrast, making objects appear in sharper detail.

Multifocal lenses

Some people have monofocal lenses. Their eyeglasses are equipped to correct just one form of vision deficiency — nearsightedness or farsightedness that may include astigmatism. Other people have multifocal lenses. Multifocal lenses combine two or more focal powers in one lens. When wearing multifocal lenses, you can shift from one focal power to another by moving your gaze to different sections of the lens. Chances are that by the time you enter your 40s, you may be using multifocal lenses.

Bifocals

As its name implies, the bifocal style combines two focal powers in one lens. The top part of the lens is adjusted for distance vision, while the lower part accommodates your close-up vision, such as for reading.

Trifocals

The trifocal lens adds a third power for an intermediate focus between your distance vision and close-up vision. The added focal power helps you clearly see objects approximately 2 to 4 feet away, such as a computer monitor or the items on a grocery store shelf.

Progressives

Unlike a trifocal lens, a progressive lens has no division lines separating the focal powers. Instead, the focal powers change smoothly as your eyes move from top to bottom. Some people report blurred vision along the sides and bottom edges of the lenses, away from the main focal points. However, newer lenses may come with less distortion. Because of the design of progressive lenses, the lens area that provides the sharpest reading is smaller than the area with bifocal or trifocal lenses.

Multifocal lenses may take some getting used to. The first step is making sure the frames are properly adjusted to fit your head. Tilt your head up and down. Your line of vision should move smoothly from one focal power to the other in both eyes at precisely the same time.

The most difficult adjustment with progressive lenses may be gauging the distance of steps, stairs and curbs when walking. When you look down at the ground with a multifocal lens, unless you tilt your head to look through the top (distance) portion of the lenses, you'll be looking through the reading portion, which will blur and distort the distance (depth) to the ground.

Frames

When looking for new glasses, you may want to begin with all of the frames on a display rack. Save yourself time and guesswork by starting with your prescription. Certain lens prescriptions work better with some frames than with others. For example, a prescription for astigmatism works well with small frames

that have rounded edges — there's less distortion from having too much lens outside your line of vision. With your prescription in hand, a skilled optician can help focus your search.

Size

Frame size can be important for your vision as well as your looks. Some eye doctors believe the frame should cover 20% to 30% of your face, with the top of the frame following the line of your eyebrows. If your frame is too large, the lenses pick up glare from overhead lights and distort your vision. If the frame is too small, your field of vision may be limited. If you need strong (thick) lenses, smaller frames help reduce the overall weight of your glasses.

Materials

Frames come in different grades of metal and plastic. Most often, you get what you pay for. If you buy the least expensive metal or plastic frame, you'll likely get a lower quality material — depending on your needs and lifestyle, that may be just fine. Thin metal frames are often the lightest, but plastic frames are usually more durable and offer better support for thick lenses.

The cheapest metal frames are made from a mixture of metals including nickel. Some frames may corrode from contact with perspiration and body oils. The more expensive metal frames made of titanium and carbon graphite are especially

NONPRESCRIPTION READING GLASSES

As you enter your 40s, you may find that you need glasses just for reading. Nonprescription reading glasses with lenses of various strengths are commonly found in pharmacies and discount stores. Reading glasses may also function when worn over contact lenses that correct for distance vision.

If your eye doctor indicated the correction you need for your reading vision, look for lenses of that focal power. Otherwise, use trial and error by holding printed material at the reading distance you prefer (typically 14 to 18 inches from your eyes) while trying different powers.

Higher powers provide more magnification and allow you to hold materials closer. Lower powers provide a focal point that's farther away. The power of the reading glasses isn't important as long as you're happy with the clarity of your vision and the distance at which you have to hold reading materials.

This general guide indicates which focal power is commonly associated with various age ranges:

Ages	Power
40 to 42	+1.00
43 to 46	+1.25
47 to 50	+1.75
51 to 54	+2.00
55 to 60	+2.25
61 and older	+2.50 or higher

You'll need prescription reading glasses if each eye requires a different power or if you need vision correction for distance. Whether you use prescription or nonprescription reading glasses, it's a good idea to see your eye doctor whenever you notice any vision changes.

durable. Beryllium, a low-cost alternative to titanium, also is lightweight, flexible and resistant to corrosion. Flexon, a titanium-based alloy, has "shape memory." You can bend and twist it, and it springs back into shape.

Plastic frames vary in their level of quality. Propionate plastic is used in cheaper frames, zyl plastic is more stylish and colorful but often brittle, and Kevlar, the same strong fiber used for military helmets, is very durable. Frames made of a resin called Optyl can be twisted around your finger and snap back into shape.

Fit

If your glasses fit correctly, they'll feel snug and secure yet won't rub behind your ears or irritate the bridge of your nose. If the frames bother you, they can be adjusted at the hinges, bridge or temples — the side arms of the frame that rest on your ears. You can also change the tilt of your glasses or adjust them to fit closer to your face.

Your nose supports about 90% of the weight of your glasses. So the nose bridge is a factor in how comfortable your glasses feel. A saddle bridge is a good choice for heavier glasses. It's a single piece of molded plastic that rides on top of your nose like a saddle, evenly spreading the weight. The most common bridge uses adjustable pads that sit on each side of your nose. Soft silicone material in the pads keeps the frames from sliding.

The temples should hook snugly around your ears and not be so thick that they block vision. Unlike standard hinges, which open to a set distance, spring hinges hold your glasses tightly to your head but allow the temples to be pulled wider so that the frames slip on or off easily.

It may take a few days to get used to new glasses. During this time, you may experience some eye ache, but the discomfort shouldn't be unbearable. If it's so painful that you can't wear the glasses, or if the pain lasts more than 2 to 3 weeks, check with your optician first. Adjusting the frames may help. Also make sure your prescription is correct. It's a good idea to have your eyeglasses fit every year or so. No matter how sturdy or cared for they are, glasses easily get out of alignment.

CONTACT LENSES

Sometimes, eyeglasses can be a nuisance. They may slide around on your nose. They get dirty when you're active, blur vision in rain, and fog up when you come inside from the cold or are wearing a face mask. They always need attention to stay in alignment. And there's the ongoing worry that some accident or mishap is going to bend them into an abstract piece of artwork.

Contact lenses are an alternative to eyeglasses. Contacts are thin, clear disks of plastic that float on the tear film that coats the cornea of your eye.

Soft contacts

Soft contact lenses are the most popular type of contact lens, both in the United States and worldwide. Soft contact lenses can be used to correct various vision problems, including:

- Nearsightedness
- Farsightedness
- Astigmatism
- Gradual age-related loss of close-up vision (presbyopia)

Soft contact lenses are made of supple plastic and conform to the shape of your eye. They're generally comfortable and tend to stay in place well, so they're a good choice if you participate in sports or lead an active lifestyle.

Soft contact lenses come in various types, including:

- **Daily wear.** Daily wear lenses are typically the least expensive option among types of soft contacts. You wear the lenses during the day and remove them each night to be cleaned and disinfected. How many days you can use a single pair of daily wear lenses varies depending on the manufacturer.
- **Extended wear.** For several consecutive days, you can keep extended wear soft contact lenses in your eyes while you sleep. But the lenses must be removed for cleaning and disinfecting at least once a week. You need to be very careful if you wear contact lenses overnight because doing so increases the risk of eye infections, even if the lenses are approved for extended wear.
- **Disposable.** Disposable lenses are generally the most expensive soft

contacts option, but they're also the most hygienic. You wear the lenses during the day and remove them at night and throw them away. The next time you want to wear contacts, you put in a new pair. You might consider disposable lenses if you wear contacts occasionally, you can't tolerate disinfecting solution or you place a high priority on convenience.

Rigid, gas permeable contacts

The gas permeable lenses available today are different from earlier hard lenses. Today's lenses are made in such a way that oxygen can pass through the rigid plastic the lens is made of, which is better for eye health and comfort.

Rigid, gas permeable lenses — some people refer to them as hard contacts — provide clear, crisp sight that can correct most vision problems. They may be appealing if you've tried soft contact lenses and been unsatisfied with the correction they provide.

Gas permeable lenses are often more breathable than are soft contact lenses, which reduces the risk of eye infections. And they may be a better option for people with irregular or uneven corneas who might not otherwise be able to wear contacts.

On the other hand, because they're highly customizable, they're more complex to fit than a soft lens. And because they're fairly rigid, they can be harder to get used to at first. It might take a few weeks for your eyes to adjust to them. They're also more likely to slip off the center of your eye than are soft contact lenses — which may lead to discomfort and blurred vision.

Gas permeable lenses must be removed for cleaning and disinfection at night. If your prescription doesn't change and you take care of your lenses, you can use the same pair for up to two or three years.

Specialized contacts

Depending on your vision needs, you might consider specialized types of contact lenses.

Hybrid contact lenses

Hybrid contact lenses feature a hard, gas permeable center surrounded by a soft outer ring. Hybrid contact lenses may be an option if you have an irregular corneal curvature (keratoconus) or you have trouble wearing regular gas permeable lenses.

Scleral contact lenses

These lenses are made from the same oxygen-permeable, rigid material as gas permeable contact lenses. They're larger than gas permeable lenses and are made to completely vault over the corneal surface. They rest entirely on the white part (sclera) of the eye. This allows them to be more comfortable than gas permeable lenses but still provide vision correction for irregular corneal surfaces.

In some cases, the cornea is so irregular that a gas permeable lens cannot sit (stabilize) on the eye. This is an ideal situation to try a scleral lens.

Scleral lenses also maintain a layer of fluid (preservative-free saline) between the back of the lens and the surface of the eye, which makes them a potential treatment for severe dry eyes. Because scleral lenses are highly customized to the eye, it may take multiple visits before the fitting is complete.

Multifocal contact lenses

Multifocal lenses, which are available in both soft and hard varieties, can correct nearsightedness, farsightedness and astigmatism in combination with presbyopia. However, it's important to keep in mind that when trying to correct for multiple distances within a small lens, clarity of vision may need to be sacrificed at one distance in order to get a better range of vision at other distances. Some people don't adapt well to these modifications.

Newer types of bifocal contact lenses offer distance correction through the peripheral part of the lens and near correction through the central part of the lens or, alternately, distance correction through the center of the lens and near correction in the peripheral part.

It's best to test them out. A trial period of wearing multifocal lenses will let you know if either style can provide you with satisfactory vision.

Tinted contact lenses

Some contact lenses are tinted, either for cosmetic reasons or therapeutic purposes — for example, to enhance your perception of color or help compensate for color blindness.

If you purchase tinted lenses, make sure they come from an eye specialist. Avoid costume or decorative contact lenses, which can damage your eyes and cause potentially serious eye infections. And never share contacts that have been worn by another individual.

Avoiding eye infections

Wearing contact lenses of any type increases the risk of a corneal infection. That's because a contact lens will reduce the amount of oxygen that reaches your cornea. Getting an eye infection doesn't need to be inevitable, however.

To prevent an infection, follow your eye doctor's instructions in caring for and using your contact lenses. In addition:

- **Practice good hygiene.** Wash, rinse and dry your hands thoroughly before handling your contacts.

MONOVISION FOR PRESBYOPIA

A treatment option for the age-related loss of close-up vision (presbyopia) is monovision therapy. With monovision contact lenses, you wear a contact lens for distance vision in your dominant eye (or no contact lens if your distance vision is fine) and a contact lens for close-up vision in your nondominant eye (or no contact lens if your near vision is fine). Your dominant eye is generally the one you use when you're aiming a camera to take a picture.

A modified monovision approach is to wear a bifocal contact lens in your nondominant eye and a contact lens set for distance vision in your dominant eye. You use both eyes for distance and one eye for reading. Your brain learns which lens to favor — depending on whether you're viewing things close or far away — so you don't have to consciously make the choice of which eye to use.

If you're considering LASIK surgery (see pages 195-200), monovision is also an approach that can be used to correct your vision. For example, if you're in your 40s and planning to use LASIK surgery to correct nearsightedness, your surgeon may offer you the option of correcting one eye for distance vision and the other for reading vision. Not everyone is able to adjust to or tolerate monovision, though, so it's wise to undergo a trial with contact lenses before opting for a permanent surgical procedure.

- **Remove your contacts before you go to sleep.** This practice applies to extended wear contacts, too. Although extended wear contacts are approved to be worn overnight, continuous use significantly increases your risk of eye infections.

- **Avoid contact with water.** Remove your contact lenses before you bathe, swim or use a hot tub. Also, never rinse your contacts with water.

- **Don't moisten your lenses with saliva.** Resist any temptation to put your lenses in your mouth to wet them.

- **Take care with contact lens solutions.** Use only commercially prepared, sterile products designed specifically for the type of contact lenses you wear — don't use water or homemade saline solution. Discard the solution in a contact lens case each time you disinfect the lenses, and don't "top off" old solution that's already in the case. Rinse the case in fresh solution, not in water, then allow the case to air dry.

- **Rub and rinse your lenses.** Gently rub your lenses when cleaning them after removal, even if you choose no-rub solution.

- **Pay attention to the expiration date.** Don't use contact solution that's past its expiration date.

- **Replace contact lenses and cases as recommended.** Follow manufacturer guidelines for replacing your contact lenses — and replace your contact lens case every 3 to 6 months.

Even with proper lens care, dry eyes can become an issue for individuals who wear contact lenses. If your eyes are itchy or red, remove your contact lenses and administer lubricating eye drops to relieve discomfort.

If your vision becomes blurry or you experience eye pain, sensitivity to light or other problems, remove your contact lenses and consult your eye doctor for prompt treatment.

REFRACTIVE SURGERY

If you're tired of putting something in your eyes or in front of your eyes to see better, you may be among the millions of people interested in refractive surgery. Refractive surgery improves vision by correcting the curvature of your cornea, which can resolve many common vision problems, such as farsightedness, nearsightedness and astigmatism. It's not as helpful for presbyopia, the decline in reading vision that usually starts in your 40s.

The popularity of refractive surgery is due in no small part to its effectiveness — the surgery really does allow many people to get rid of their glasses or contacts. Refractive surgery may be especially attractive if you work in a dusty job and wear contact lenses, or if you're constantly going indoors and out-of-doors in cold weather and dealing with foggy glasses. When swimming or water-skiing, eyeglasses and contact lenses can be impractical or impossible to wear.

However, refractive surgery may not always be the best option for correcting your vision. It can produce serious side effects, some of which are described on pages 199-200.

There are several different types of refractive surgery. LASIK surgery — short for laser-assisted in-situ keratomileusis — is the most common type. Other types of refractive surgery, including procedures known as PRK, LASEK and SMILE, use similar technologies but with slight variations that may be more suitable for correcting specific problems.

LASIK

With the knowledge collected from years of experience and many critical advances in technology, the outcome of LASIK surgery continues to improve. But complications associated with LASIK still exist, and the procedure isn't always covered by insurance. Before you schedule LASIK, talk to your eye doctor and make sure you fully understand the procedure and its benefits and risks.

Unlike many sight-threatening eye diseases, refractive errors aren't progressive in themselves, and they may improve over time. Some doctors, therefore, are reluctant to endorse a relatively invasive eye surgery such as LASIK to correct nearsightedness or farsightedness. Their reasoning is that your eyes are basically healthy and your vision can be improved with less risky measures, such as eyeglasses or contact lenses.

Refractive surgery is usually an elective surgery, which means it isn't vital to your health and well-being. For this reason, Medicare and most insurance companies don't cover the cost of the procedure.

Preparing for LASIK

For your eyes to accurately focus light coming into them, three elements must

INSIDE OUT?

Soft contact lenses sometimes turn inside out as you handle them. Putting them in your eye this way causes irritation and eye watering. In fact, if your eye hurts as soon as you insert a lens, it's very likely the contact is inside out.

There are two ways to check whether a contact is inside out before putting it in your eye. The first way is to place the lens on the tip of your finger and look closely at the rim. If the rim is pointing straight up like the edge of a bowl, it's OK. If the edge is flared out, the lens is likely inside out.

A second way is to put the lens on a crease line in the palm of your hand and gently cup your hand. If the edges roll neatly toward each other, like they're forming a tiny taco shell, the lens is right side out. If they start to fold backward, away from the center, the lens is turned inside out.

be precisely balanced and coordinated — the shape of the cornea, the condition of the natural lens and the length of the eyeball. The cornea and the lens bend all of the light entering the front of the eye to a precise focal point.

In a normally shaped eye, that point should create a sharp image directly on the retina. Nearsightedness or farsightedness occurs when the combined focusing power of the cornea and the lens converges at a point that falls in front of or behind the retina.

LASIK eye surgery improves vision by changing the curvature of the cornea to adjust for any misalignment. It shifts the focal point more precisely onto your retina.

A good surgical outcome depends on the careful evaluation of your eyes before you undergo LASIK surgery or a similar procedure. Your eye surgeon can help determine if you're a good candidate for surgery.

To assess your readiness for LASIK surgery, your eye surgeon will take a detailed medical and surgical history and conduct a comprehensive eye examination. During the eye examination, your surgeon will evaluate your vision and look for signs of eye infections, inflammation, dry eyes, large pupils, high eye pressure or other eye conditions.

Your surgeon will also assess which areas of your cornea need reshaping in order to correct your vision problem. Imaging technology known as corneal topography

creates a highly detailed surface map of your cornea — similar to a topographical map — noting its shape, contour, thickness and any irregularities. Theoretically, the more detailed the measurements of your cornea, the more accurately your eye surgeon can evaluate problems and remove corneal tissue.

If you regularly wear contact lenses, you'll need to switch to glasses for a few weeks before your appointment with the surgeon. Contact lenses can slightly distort the shape of your cornea, which may lead to an inaccurate measurement of the cornea and a poor surgical outcome.

Skip eye makeup and eye cream for several days before your surgery. Your surgeon may instruct you to clean your eyelashes prior to surgery to remove debris and minimize your risk of infection. You'll also want to arrange for someone to drive you home after the procedure. That's because you may be feeling the effects of medication given before surgery and your vision may still be blurry.

The LASIK procedure

Laser-assisted in-situ keratomileusis (LASIK) is performed using an excimer laser. This laser is a specialized device that's programmed to remove a precise amount of tissue from your cornea in a clearly defined pattern.

The excimer laser doesn't cut or burn tissue. It emits a cold (nonthermal) energy that controls the amount of tissue removed from the corneal surface, one microscopic layer at a time. The procedure is carefully planned out beforehand based on the results of your eye examination and medical imaging. Often, surgery can be performed on both eyes on the same day.

Prior to surgery, you'll receive anesthetic eye drops to numb your eye during the

procedure, which helps ensure you'll experience little pain. You may also be given medicine to help you relax.

LASIK surgery usually takes less than 30 minutes. You lie on your back in a reclining chair for the procedure. After numbing drops are placed in your eye, a special instrument is put in place to hold your eyelids open. A suction ring is positioned

CORNEAL TOPOGRAPHY

To prepare for LASIK surgery, your eye surgeon uses special imaging that precisely maps the shape and contour of your cornea. This image will guide the surgeon's work in reshaping your cornea with an excimer laser.

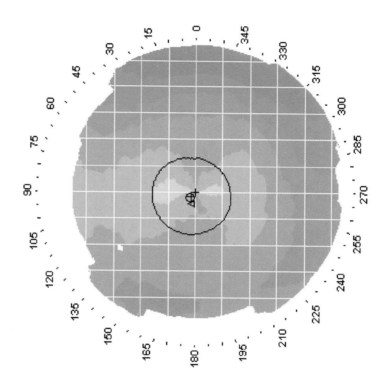

on the eye, which may apply slight pressure, and your vision may dim a little.

As the surgical procedure is taking place, you'll be asked to focus on a point of light. Staring at this light helps keep your eye fixed while the laser reshapes your cornea.

LASIK SURGERY

To begin the LASIK procedure, your surgeon uses a laser or special blade to cut a circular flap on the top layer of your cornea. Folding back this flap allows access to deeper layers of tissue (left). A laser reshapes the exposed tissue, making it flatter or steeper depending on your needs for corrected vision (center). When reshaping is complete, the corneal flap is repositioned over the treated area and allowed to heal on its own (right).

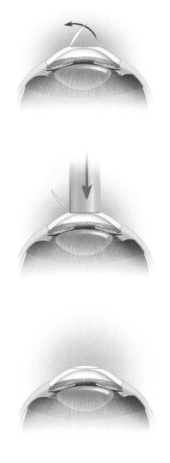

To begin, your surgeon will cut a circular flap of tissue from the center of your cornea. This may be done with a type of laser called a femtosecond laser or, occasionally, a mechanical device called a microkeratome.

The flap, which is still hinged to the cornea, is about the size and shape of a contact lens. It is folded out of the way,

allowing the surgeon to reshape corneal tissue underneath it with an excimer laser — removing one microscopic layer at a time. You may detect a distinct odor as the laser removes corneal tissue. After the reshaping of your cornea is complete, the flap is folded back into place and usually heals without stitches.

Immediately after LASIK surgery, your eyes may burn or itch and be watery. Your vision may be blurry. You may still feel the effects of the medication given to you before surgery.

You may need to take pain medication for several hours after the procedure. You may also need to wear a shield over your eye at night until it heals.

Typically, you're able to see afterward but your vision won't necessarily be clear right away. It usually takes about 2 to 3 months after surgery before your eyes heal and your vision stabilizes.

You'll likely see your surgeon again shortly after surgery and at regular intervals for the next few months. In general, you have a very good chance of achieving 20/25 vision or better after refractive surgery. Your chances for improved vision are based, in part, on how good your vision was before surgery.

It may be a few weeks before you can start to use cosmetics or creams around your eyes again. You might also have to wait several weeks before resuming strenuous contact sports, swimming or using hot tubs.

Reasons to not choose LASIK

Certain risk factors may rule out LASIK surgery as an option for correcting vision problems. You shouldn't have this surgery if you:

POSSIBLE RISKS

As with any type of surgery, refractive surgery carries risks, including:

- **Undercorrection.** If the laser removes too little tissue from your cornea, your vision may not be as clear as you were hoping for. You may need another surgery to remove more tissue.
- **Overcorrection.** It's possible that the laser will remove too much tissue from your cornea. An overcorrection can be more difficult to fix than an undercorrection.
- **Astigmatism.** Astigmatism may result from uneven tissue healing or uneven tissue removal from your cornea. The development may require additional surgery.
- **Glare, halos and double vision.** After surgery you may have difficulty seeing at night or in low-light conditions, such as fog. You may notice glare, halos around bright lights or double vision. Sometimes these symptoms can be treated with corticosteroid eye drops or by wearing mild prescription eyeglasses while driving at night. Other times, a second surgery is required.
- **Dry eyes.** LASIK surgery causes a temporary decrease in tear production. As your eyes heal after surgery, they may feel unusually dry. You'll likely need to administer eye drops during this time.
- **Flap problems.** Folding back or removing the flap from your eye during surgery can cause complications, including infection, tearing and swelling. In some cases, the flap may wrinkle or become dislodged before healing is complete.

• **Have a condition that may impair your ability to heal.** Certain diseases that affect your immune system may impair your ability to heal after the surgery. The risks of incomplete healing, infection and other complications are increased if you have an autoimmune disease, such as rheumatoid arthritis, or an immunodeficiency disease, such as the human immunodeficiency virus (HIV). Taking an immunosuppressive drug also disqualifies you from having this surgery.

• **Have persistent dry eyes.** Conditions that causes dry eyes, including Sjögren's syndrome, may impair healing.

• **Have an extremely uneven corneal surface or an otherwise abnormally shaped cornea.** Deep-set eyes or thin corneas also may make the surgery more difficult.

• **Have unstable vision.** If your vision fluctuates or is progressively worsening, you may not be eligible for LASIK surgery.

• **Are pregnant or breastfeeding.** These can cause vision to fluctuate and make the outcome of surgery less certain.

Refractive surgery may also not be a good choice if:

• **It jeopardizes your career.** Some jobs, in which very precise vision is required, may prohibit certain refractive procedures.

• **Cost is an issue.** Although refractive surgery is becoming less expensive, it's still a significant cost and most insurance companies don't pay for it.

• **You have a high refractive error in your prescription.** If you have severe nearsightedness — a strong prescription — the surgery may not produce acceptable results.

• **You have a low refractive error in your prescription.** If you only need to wear contacts or glasses some of the time, improvement from the surgery may not be worth the risk of complications.

• **You have large pupils.** Refractive surgery on people prone to having large pupils in dim light can result in debilitating symptoms such as glare, halos and ghost images.

• **You actively participate in contact sports.** If you frequently participate in boxing, martial arts or other activities in which blows to the face and eyes are a normal occurrence, refractive surgery may not be in your best interest. Another procedure called PRK may be a better option.

OTHER REFRACTIVE PROCEDURES

If you're not a good candidate for LASIK surgery, your surgeon may recommend another type of refractive surgery. There are a variety of options.

Photorefractive keratectomy

Photorefractive keratectomy (PRK) is sometimes used if you have a low to moderate degree of nearsightedness or farsightedness, or if you have nearsightedness combined with astigmatism. Most people have surgery on both eyes on the same day.

During PRK, your surgeon uses an excimer laser to remove the outermost surface of the cornea and re-sculpt its curvature. Unlike LASIK surgery, PRK doesn't involve creating a flap of corneal tissue that must be repositioned after the surgery. Instead, the exposed surface of your cornea naturally repairs itself, often assisted by a temporary contact lens worn as a bandage over your eye for three or four days after surgery.

You may have eye pain for a few days until your cornea heals. It generally takes up to a week for your eye to regenerate the surface tissue. It may take 3 to 6 months for your vision to improve completely.

PRK is performed less commonly than is LASIK, largely because healing after LASIK tends to be more predictable and usually involves less discomfort. However, thanks to improved technology, PRK is experiencing a bit of a rebound. With PRK, healing takes longer but there's generally less risk because there are no flap complications to worry about.

Laser-assisted subepithelial keratectomy

With laser-assisted subepithelial keratectomy (LASEK), your eye surgeon makes a very shallow incision on the thin, top layer of the cornea (epithelium) with a special cutting instrument. An alcohol solution is placed on the epithelium to loosen it so the ultrathin flap can be peeled back. The flap is pushed aside to access deeper layers that need reshaping.

The shaping process performed during surgery is done with a special cutting

device, the same instrument used for PRK and LASIK. After the cornea is reshaped, the epithelial flap is smoothed back into place and a contact bandage is placed on your eye to promote healing, similar to the PRK procedure.

If you have a very thin cornea, you might be a good candidate for LASEK because the procedure allows your eye surgeon to remove very little of the cornea, leaving its structural integrity intact. People who play contact sports or work in a

PRK SURGERY

Unlike LASIK, with the PRK procedure an eye surgeon does not create a protective flap. Instead, the surgeon works directly on the outermost layer of the cornea using an excimer laser, reshaping the surface to correct vision.

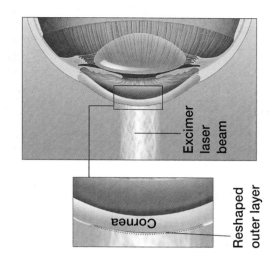

Excimer laser beam

Cornea

Reshaped outer layer

profession that carries an increased risk of eye trauma also may benefit from LASIK, because flap complications are fewer and less serious than with LASIK.

However, because the corneal flap is so thin, it may dislodge more easily, which can cause eye pain and require additional surgery. LASEK surgery can be done on both eyes on the same day.

Epi-LASIK

A technique called epi-LASIK is similar to LASIK and LASEK. The epi-LASIK flap is very similar to the thin flap created with LASEK surgery. The difference is in the instruments and techniques used in creating the flap. Also, unlike LASEK, the epi-LASIK procedure doesn't involve an alcohol solution that's applied to the eye. For this reason, epi-LASIK may cause less eye pain and haziness.

SMILE

SMILE, which stands for small incision lenticule extraction, is a newer technology. A femtosecond laser is used to isolate a small amount of cornea (a lenticle), which is then removed through a tiny incision.

An advantage of this procedure is that it involves a small incision rather than a flap. Its disadvantages are that it's newer and it cannot yet correct as wide a range of nearsightedness, farsightedness and astigmatism conditions as can LASIK or PRK.

Implantable lenses

With this procedure, special corrective lenses (phakic intraocular lenses) are surgically inserted into the eye to improve vision. The technology works by placing an implantable lens in front of the natural lens.

One of the advantages of implantable lenses is that they can correct high degrees of nearsightedness, farsightedness and astigmatism — conditions that limit the use of other surgical procedures. For people with moderate to severe nearsightedness, phakic intraocular lenses reduce the risk of complications after surgery while providing better vision compared with correction from laser surgery.

Implantable lenses are relatively new, though. Scientists are working on improving the lenses and surgical techniques. Possible complications, such as cataracts, increased pressure within the eye and damage to the cornea over time, remain a concern.

Intracorneal ring segments

Refractive surgery techniques can treat specialized conditions. For example, intracorneal ring segments (ICRS) have been used to treat mild nearsightedness but are more often used to treat keratoconus. This is a condition in which the cornea becomes progressively thinner and is distorted into a cone shape, creating vision problems and making it difficult to wear contact lenses.

During the procedure, a small incision is made in the cornea, and two crescent-shaped plastic rings are placed on the cornea's outer edge. The rings help restore a more normal shape to the cornea and are less invasive than a corneal transplant. The rings can also be removed if necessary.

BEST RESULTS

The goal of refractive surgery is to achieve functional vision, which refers to your ability to do most daily tasks without corrective lenses. More than 8 out of 10 people who've undergone refractive surgery no longer need to use their glasses or contact lenses for the majority of functional activities.

In some specific situations, however, such as driving at night, you may still need corrective lenses to achieve your best vision.

Your surgical outcome depends on your specific refractive error and other factors. People with a low grade of nearsightedness tend to have the most success with refractive surgery. People with a high degree of nearsightedness or farsightedness along with astigmatism have less predictable results and are more likely to need a second surgery (enhancement surgery) to correct lingering focusing difficulties.

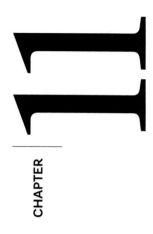

11

Living with low vision

Throughout this book you've learned how various eye diseases are diagnosed and treated. While prompt treatment may stop or lessen damage to your eyes, it may not restore your vision back to normal. If your vision loss makes daily tasks difficult to perform, you have low vision.

Vision loss can be frightening and overwhelming; the thought of losing independence can create anxiety and depression, but know that you are not alone. Vision rehabilitation can help you learn about vision loss, find adaptive tools, and discover your coping skills and strengths. You can live well with low vision.

Low vision affects everyone differently. For one person, it makes reading difficult. For another, driving is impossible. For yet another, cooking is a problem.

Permanent vision loss may stem from a single disease, such as macular degeneration or glaucoma, or it may be the cumulative result of several conditions, such as diabetes, high blood pressure and eye disease. Vision loss can also result from serious eye injuries, birth defects or neurological conditions, such as a brain injury or stroke. The effects of low vision may range from mild to severe.

Living with vision loss isn't an easy experience for anyone. It can affect many facets of your life, including your job, social life and leisure activities, as well as your self-confidence and mental health.

Rehabilitation can help you adjust to vision loss. A low-vision specialist can help you incorporate optical technology into your daily routine. He or she can also provide tips and strategies to make the most of your remaining vision. The goal is to help you continue living independently, while maintaining your quality of life.

VISION REHABILITATION

Many people with low vision believe there's little that can be done for them. It's true that lost vision can't be restored, but many types of vision loss can be managed through vision rehabilitation, sometimes referred to as low-vision rehabilitation.

What is vision rehabilitation? It's a combination of testing, specialized training and counseling services that help you develop special skills that allow you to continue taking part in day-to-day activities. While vision rehabilitation can't restore vision, it can improve your ability to function in life by providing you the skills you need to maintain a greater degree of independence.

Vision rehabilitation starts with an assessment by a low-vision specialist — an ophthalmologist or optometrist with training in low vision. This specialist can determine your vision capabilities and develop a plan to achieve your vision goals. He or she may also work with other health care professionals, such as social workers, rehabilitation therapists and occupational therapists, to maximize your remaining vision.

You may be asked to create a complete history of your vision. This history includes how long you've had low vision

and how it affects your everyday life. You may be asked to describe tasks that are causing you frustration, as well as those tasks you would like to be able to perform.

The specialist will perform tests to evaluate which low-vision aids may help you. Options may include eyeglasses, magnifiers, telescopes, electronic and technological devices, as well as nonoptical devices such as reading stands, lamps and writing templates.

Testing is not just a trial-and-error process, although sometimes it may seem that way. Often, testing must be done over several visits, as this process takes time. It can be tiresome. But the entire process is designed to maximize your vision and achieve your goals.

Once a specialist determines the best aids for you, he or she may develop a program to help you learn how to effectively use the devices. If you've tried magnifiers bought at a store or online and they don't help, don't worry. They probably aren't the correct magnification for you.

Training may be carried out by an eye specialist or by another professional, such as a vision rehabilitation specialist or occupational therapist. Training is important. Although low-vision aids may seem simple, if they're not used properly, they won't help you achieve your goals. The process is similar to rehabilitation for someone who has experienced an injury or a stroke and may need rehabilitation to relearn how to do specific tasks.

DEFINING LOW VISION

Low vision is loss of eyesight that cannot be corrected with eyeglasses, medications or surgery. It may include the loss of central vision, peripheral vision, contrast sensitivity or depth perception.

The degree of low vision — based on the level of vision in the better eye with the best possible corrective lens — is often categorized as follows:

Mild low vision: 20/30 to 20/60

Moderate low vision: 20/70 to 20/160

Severe low vision: 20/200 or worse

Profound low vision: 20/500 to 20/1,000

Near-total vision loss: Worse than 20/1,000

Total visual impairment: No light perception

There are additional categories of visual impairment based on the loss of peripheral vision.

In the United States, anyone with vision that can't be corrected to better than 20/200 in the best eye, or who has 20 degrees or less of visual field remaining, is considered legally blind. Most people who are legally blind actually have some remaining sight and can learn to make good use of it with vision rehabilitation. Few people are completely blind.

It's important to note that your degree of vision loss — or category — doesn't necessarily correlate with how much low vision will interfere with your daily activities. Some people with mild to moderate low vision may experience a lot of difficulty, and some with severe low vision don't have any real problems. No matter what your degree of loss, make sure your eye specialist understands how much your vision loss is hampering your daily activities.

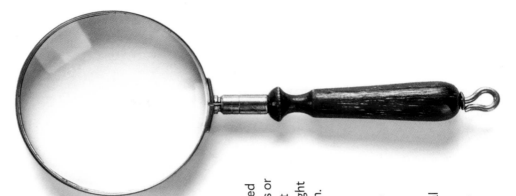

Vision rehabilitation generally focuses on three main areas:

- Independent living skills
- Orientation and mobility training
- Technological advances and electronic devices

Your low-vision specialist will work closely with you and tailor your program to meet your everyday living needs, based on your level of vision loss.

INDEPENDENT LIVING SKILLS

With low vision, you may need to relearn how to perform essential skills in a

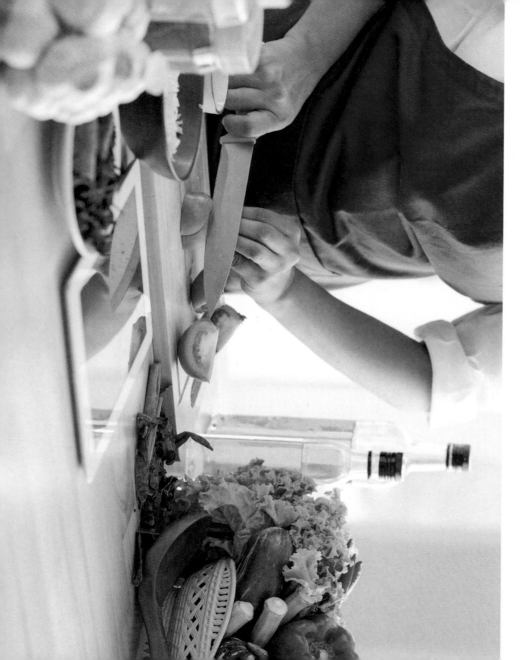

slightly different way. A wide range of basic tasks are covered in vision rehabilitation therapy, such as using the telephone, managing your money and making your home safer. Various low-vision websites offer many great tips, but here are a few suggestions to get you started.

Personal care

Being responsible for cleaning and grooming yourself is an important part of daily life. Feeling good about how you look can boost your self-esteem and keep you determined to overcome difficulties associated with low vision.

Here are tips to help you look your best:

- Find a hairstyle you like that's simple and easy to care for.
- Purchase shampoo, conditioner, body wash and other toiletries in bottles of different sizes and shapes so that you can easily tell them apart in the shower.
- Learn to apply makeup using your sense of touch. A rehabilitation specialist can help you learn to do this.
- Use rubber bands or adhesive bump dots to differentiate similar versions of the same item, such as lipstick shades. For example, put one rubber band around the pink lipstick shade, two rubber bands around the red shade and no rubber bands around the coral shade.
- Use colored or striped toothpaste that contrasts with the white bristles on your toothbrush. That should help make it easier for you to get the paste on the brush. Hold the toothpaste cap in your hand or pocket so that you don't lose it.
- For shaving safety, try using an electric razor.
- Hang large-print labels on your clothes to identify the item color. Note BR for brown, B for black and R for red on the label. You can also pin a label to the front of the item.
- Organize clothing into matching outfits with the help of a friend or relative. For example, hang a coordinating pair of pants, shirt and tie on one hanger.

Cooking

There's no need to fear the kitchen just because you have low vision. You can learn to cook just as well as a person with normal sight. It starts by honing your senses: Feel the vibration of boiling water on the kettle handle. Hear the pop of frying food to know it's browning. Learn the smell of something that's fully cooked.

Also try these techniques:

- Store utensils, pots and pans, spices, and other cooking items in obvious locations, and always return them to the places where you found them. Smell spices before you use them.
- Look for adaptive versions of common kitchen equipment, such as large-print measuring cups, talking kitchen timers, electronic liquid level indicators and long oven mitts that cover your arms.
- Organize food items in your pantry in a familiar manner. To help distinguish between similar items, have a friend or family member mark the item in big letters with a dark, felt-tip pen. You can also use the rubber band system — for example, no band for canned tomatoes, one band for canned black beans and two bands for canned chickpeas.
- Install under-the-counter lighting at locations where you prepare food.
- Mark the frequently used settings on appliance knobs and dials, using bump dots or drops of glue or nail polish. On your oven, for example, mark the "off" position and every 100 degrees of temperature.
- Use a cutting board that contrasts with the color of the food item you're preparing.
- Take advantage of cooking shortcuts. Use frozen vegetables or pre-cut varieties instead of chopping them yourself. Ask the butcher to cube a piece of meat for you.

- Use slow cookers, bread machines and other appliances that simplify the cooking process.
- Set a timer to remind you to turn off the stove or other electrical appliances.
- Use a sturdy pizza cutter instead of a knife for slicing sandwiches and other foods.

Using the telephone

Operating your home phone, work phone or cellphone can be difficult if you have trouble seeing the correct numbers to press or dial. Here are some strategies that can help:

- Have a light by your phone to help you see your phone and the dial pad.
- Use a large-print number template on top of your existing home or work telephone so that you can see the numbers more easily.
- Buy a voice-activated telephone or programmable telephone for use at home. A voice-activated phone allows you to dial preprogrammed numbers by simply speaking the name of the person you're planning to call into your receiver. A programmable telephone allows you to dial frequently used numbers with the touch of one button.
- Use a smartphone with built-in accessibility features that allow you to enlarge text, zoom in on the screen or increase contrast.
- Most smartphones have the capability for voice command. You can verbally instruct your phone to call someone. Use this feature.
- Check out phone apps designed for people with low vision, such as magnifiers, text-to-speech features, artificial intelligence to identify colors and objects, and so forth. You may need someone who is sighted to help you locate these features and teach you how to use them.
- Check out crowd assistance apps on your smartphone. These apps connect individuals with low vision to sighted volunteers or professional guides via live video calls. For example, if you need help reading the turkey thermometer, the guide person on your video call can help.

Managing money

Identifying the correct values of coins and currency can be a problem if your vision is limited. Writing checks and paying bills also can be frustrating. Try these tips:

- When making purchases, consider using a debit card or credit card so that you don't need to sort coins and bills. This also provides a permanent record of how much you were charged for the transaction.
- If paying bills is a challenge, ask your bank about online banking and automatic payments for recurring bills. You can also pay many bills by phone.
- If you write a lot of checks, find out if your bank offers large-print checks or checks printed with raised lines. Also consider check guides. These plastic templates fit over a standard check and include cutouts for where you need to write information — such as the date, amount of purchase and your signature.
- There are many time-tested techniques for identifying coins and cash, such as

folding bills of different denominations into different shapes and learning to recognize coins by their size, texture and thickness. A vision rehabilitation therapist can teach you a variety of techniques.

- Use a talking calculator. This type of calculator announces the keys you've just pressed and reports the results.

Taking medications

It's important that you take all medications and supplements properly. Whether you're taking daily vitamins, over-the-counter medications or prescription pills, follow these tips for properly identifying your medications and ensuring that you take them safely:

- Learn to recognize the medications you take regularly by noting their shape and size.
- Ask your pharmacist for large-print labels on your prescription medication containers, as well as large-print instructions. You can also ask the pharmacist to put prescription medications into containers of different sizes so that you can easily tell them apart.
- Buy a pill organizer with a beeping or vibrating alarm to alert you when it's time for the next dose. Other options include asking your pharmacist about the availability of blister cards or to wrap rubber bands around your containers equal to the number of daily doses. This will help you remember if you've taken the right amount.

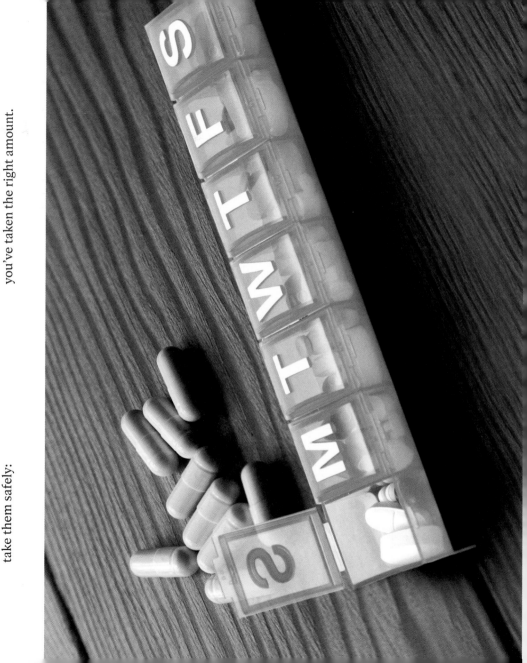

- Use a weekly pill organizer. Pill organizers contain boxes for the days of the week, and you can buy one with large-print labels or tactile marks. A friend or family member can help you fill the organizer each week. Then, you can confidently take the pills every day.
- Use special markings to differentiate the medications that you keep at home, including vitamins, pain relievers or prescription medications. You can use adhesive bump dots, rubber bands, color-coded labels, or drops of glue or nail polish.

Creating a safe environment

Home safety is important for every home. When you have low vision, it's especially critical that you organize your surroundings and eliminate potential hazards that could lead to injuries or falls:

LIGHT UP YOUR LIFE

Most adults need more light for close-up tasks as they get older. If you have low vision, you'll need good lighting when you use low-vision aids. Good lighting also helps you avoid obstructions and trip hazards in your pathway:

- Keep the level of lighting consistent throughout your house, even if that means keeping some house lights on during the day. Consistent lighting can minimize shadows and bright spots.
- When reading or doing detail work, don't face the windows. Position yourself so that the windows are behind you or to the side.
- Use an adjustable lamp for reading or doing other close-up work. Two of the best options are a gooseneck lamp or a lamp with a swivel arm that can be raised or lowered. Position the lamp about 4 to 8 inches from your reading material, but slightly off to the side to reduce glare.
- Direct your light source over the shoulder of the eye that has your best vision.
- Install lighting under shelves and cupboards in kitchen, study and work areas to increase visibility.
- Wear a visor or hat with a wide brim indoors to block annoying overhead light.

Reducing surface glare in your home is just as important as improving your lighting, because glare can make it difficult for you to see. If possible, choose furnishings with a flat or matte finish, rather than a glossy finish. Cover shiny surfaces, such as a polished table, with a cloth. Place a dark piece of construction paper behind your reading material to reduce glare when you read. Also, consider window coverings that reduce glare, such as miniblinds.

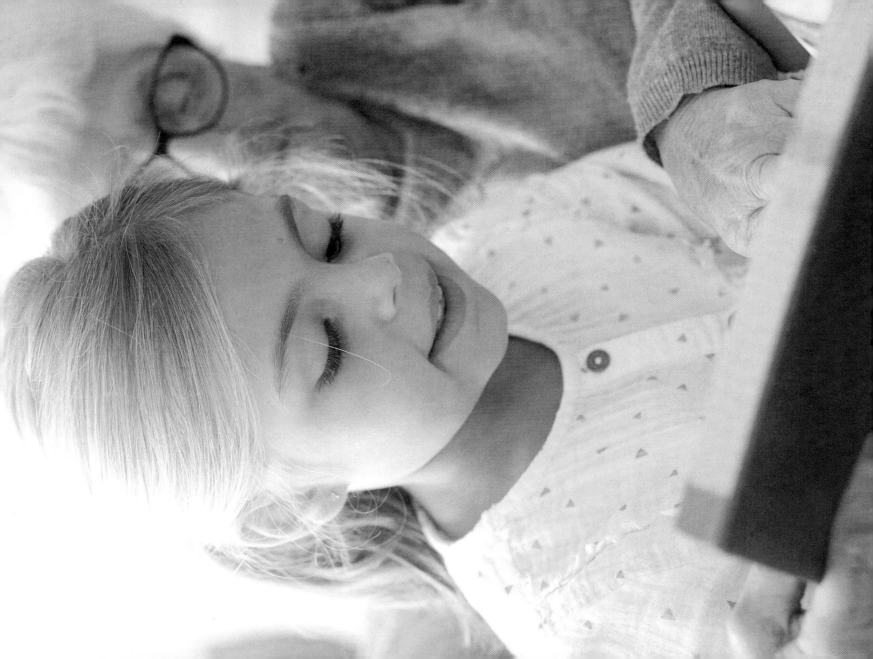

- Increase the lighting in your home (see page 212).

- Arrange furniture so that sharp corners and edges don't interfere with or obstruct normal traffic patterns throughout the house.

- Eliminate throw rugs and other tripping hazards, such as loose extension cords. Keep the floor clear of shoes, clothing, newspapers and other items.

- Raised door thresholds and steps can be difficult to see. Use safety tape or contrasting paint to highlight these areas, especially top and bottom steps. Make sure your stairways are well lit.

- Install sturdy banisters or grab rails on stairs and in the bathroom.

- Close closet doors and cupboard drawers as soon as you're done using them. Doors and drawers left partially open are frequent causes of accidents.

- Install an intercom or specialized doorbell at your front door so that visitors can easily identify themselves when they arrive.

- Install wireless sensor lights throughout the house so that your pathway is always illuminated, especially when you return home in the evening. A less expensive option is to place an automatic night light in your entry area.

- Mark the "start" position on the dials of your washing machine and dishwasher with bump dots or some other labeling technique. Do the same for comfortable temperature settings on your thermostat. Consider installing a large-print or talking thermostat.

- Store similarly shaped containers, such as spray cans of insect repellent and air freshener, in separate locations. Mark each container to help identify it.

- Don't ignore the exterior of your home. Mark the edges of outdoor steps with paint or duct tape in a contrasting color. Place low-voltage lighting and contrasting plants along paths and walkways. Remove trip hazards from the yard.

ORIENTATION AND MOBILITY TRAINING

It's not uncommon for people with low vision to be reluctant to travel outside of their home, due to safety concerns and the fear of getting lost. However, giving into this fear is a major blow to independence and can have a negative impact on quality of life.

That's why orientation and mobility training is a key component of vision rehabilitation. This type of training focuses on strategies for feeling more secure and confident while outside your home. Orientation refers to your ability to know where you are and where you want to go. Mobility refers to your ability to get there safely and efficiently.

You may learn to get around safely by using your remaining vision or the assistance of another person (sighted guide), a white cane or a guide dog. Training may be provided by a certified orientation and mobility specialist or by an experienced health care professional.

Using your remaining vision

If you want to rely on your own eyesight to travel about safely, your vision needs to be good enough to react to the people, animals and vehicles moving around you. And you must be able to see the dangers posed by curbs, stairs, walls, fences, posts, holes and other obstacles in your pathway.

A certified specialist can teach you specific methods for moving about safely, making it possible for you to walk around your neighborhood or catch a bus to go downtown. You may learn to use a combination of senses to know where you are. You may learn methods to cross streets by analyzing traffic patterns. You can learn how to find your destination by using landmarks and compass directions. As part of your training, you may also plan ahead for situations when you get disoriented or need to change your route.

Sighted guide

If you're outside of familiar surroundings, you may find it faster and easier to travel with someone who doesn't have vision problems who can act as your guide. However, it's best to learn how to do this properly. Holding hands with your guide or resting your hand on his or her shoulder isn't the best way — this can lead to accidents.

During vision rehabilitation, you can learn how to walk safely and effectively with a guide. In general, it's best if your guide walks about half a step in front of you, while you hold the guide's arm just above the elbow. That way, you're better able to feel and follow the guide's movements.

Your guide can announce changes in the terrain, such as curbs and steps. But you should still pay attention to your surroundings and look or listen for cues that help orient you.

An orientation and mobility specialist can teach you and your guide additional traveling techniques and signals, such as how to go through doorways or navigate narrow spaces. These techniques take practice, so it's a good idea to identify a small group of close family members or friends to be trained as regular guides.

White cane

You may not like the idea of using a white cane, but it may provide you with freedom to do the things you love to do. You can use a cane to detect — or verify — obstacles in front of you, such as steps, curbs and uneven pavement.

A white cane is also a useful communication tool that lets people know that you don't see well. The color of the cane alerts passersby to use caution and to not walk in front of you. And it provides a simple explanation if you accidentally bump into someone.

Canes come in different styles — some can be folded to fit into a coat pocket or purse. Canes may be ordered online or through catalogs, but it's best to be fitted for a cane by an orientation and mobility specialist. You want it to be long enough to give you reaction time and distance to prevent an injury, but not too long so that the cane is clumsy and difficult to use. As a rule of thumb, the cane should extend from the middle of your chest to the floor, and possibly a little longer.

Guide dog

A guide dog is another type of mobility aid. Similar to a sighted guide, a guide dog can be your surrogate eyes — surveying the environment, leading you around obstacles and warning you of potential hazards. Many people with limited vision find a guide dog to be a great asset as well as a wonderful companion.

Of course, you need to be willing to care for the dog properly. This includes giving your guide dog an opportunity to practice his or her skills daily. Guide dogs will lose their skills if they're not used regularly, so they're not a good solution for someone who only goes outside the house every once in a while.

It's important to remember that a dog can't do it all. Even if you plan to use a guide dog to assist you in your daily travels, developing your mobility and orientation skills is still important.

ASSISTIVE DEVICES AND EMERGING TECHNOLOGY

A wide array of devices can help you remain actively involved in daily life. Options range from inexpensive talking clocks to more expensive video magnifiers. The devices that you feel may benefit you depend on your vision problems, lifestyle needs and comfort level with using various technologies. A member of your rehabilitation team can help you narrow your choices.

Assistive devices

Assistive devices are designed to help you use your remaining vision more effectively. They're frequently used in conjunction with regular prescription eyeglasses. Assistive devices include magnifiers for close-up work and telescopes for distance vision.

Magnifiers

Magnifiers come in many styles, shapes, sizes and different degrees of power. Traditional hand-held and stand magnifiers allow you to read printed materials or work with objects positioned at a normal distance from your eyes. A hand-held magnifier may be carried with you for reading price tags, labels and restaurant menus. Some magnifiers are small enough to fit in your pocket.

However, a hand-held device isn't very practical for reading longer texts, such as a book, because you have to hold the lens at a steady distance from the reading material, which can be exhausting to your arms. Stand magnifiers are better for this task. They can be adjusted at a fixed distance directly above the object that you're looking at.

Magnifying eyeglasses are another option. These eyeglasses contain a lens that's stronger than regular prescription

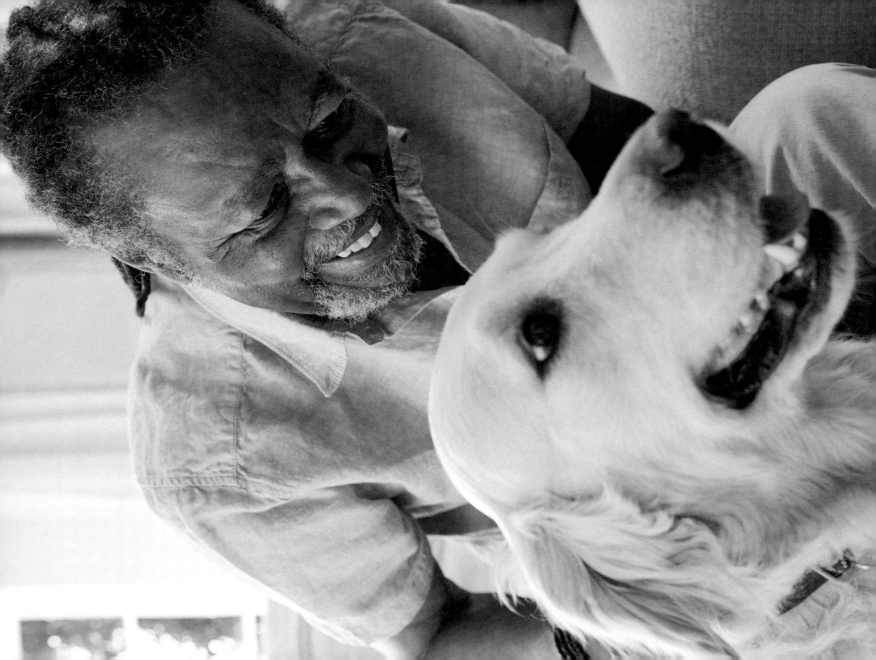

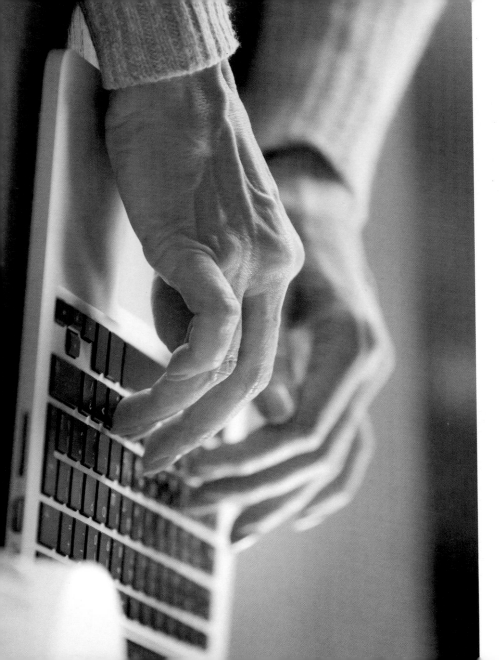

eyeglasses. Because of the strong power, you'll have to hold reading material much closer than normal. Magnifying eyeglasses help free your hands for other tasks, such as holding a book comfortably.

Whenever you use any kind of magnifier, use plenty of light for best vision.

Telescopes

Conventional magnifying lenses are intended for close-up work. They don't help you see better at a distance — even objects that are just across the room. A telescope magnifies objects in the distance, but at the expense of a greatly narrowed field of vision.

Hand-held telescopes are best for short-term use, such as reading bus numbers, store signs and street names. An eyeglass-mounted system is better for long-term use, for example, when you're at an outdoor sporting event or a concert.

Some telescopes you focus manually, while others are autofocus. Autofocus telescopes adjust focus automatically as you change the direction of your gaze, such as switching from a far-distance to intermediate-distance object.

Emerging technology

There have been many advances in technology in recent years, making it difficult to keep up with all the new devices and opportunities within the low-vision world. Ask a member of your health care team to refer you to a technology specialist who can help you explore all of the options.

Video magnifiers

A video magnifier — also referred to as a closed-circuit television system — provides much greater magnification than does a traditional magnifier. This device uses a video camera to project text or images onto a monitor or screen. Depending on the model you choose, the screen may be the size of a credit card or a computer monitor. Video magnifiers can be used to read books, newspapers, menus or labels and to look at photographs.

You can opt for a powerful video magnifier mounted on a permanent or portable stand or a hand-held system that fits in your pocket. Both work in the same way: You pass the material you want to read or look at under the camera. The camera magnifies the object and displays it on the monitor. You can also purchase video magnifiers that connect to your computer or laptop, allowing you to adjust the magnification to a size that allows you to see. You can adjust the color, brightness, contrast and background of the screen to suit your needs.

Text-to-speech technology

Instead of magnifying text onto a screen, these devices scan text and read it aloud to you. They can take words on the screen of a computer or tablet or another similar device and convert them into audio.

You place printed text under the scanning device or point to the text and an internal camera scans the print and then reads it aloud with a synthetic voice. The device can read almost anything that's printed, but it doesn't work with handwritten material. You can use the text-to-speech system by itself, or you can connect it to a computer or tablet. There are also smartphone apps that allow you to use the same technology with your cellphone.

Software programs

A magnifying software program can magnify all text that appears on your computer screen, making it easier for you to read documents, email and information that you find on the internet. Some programs may have expanded capabilities to help make it easier to use the computer. When you install a synthetic voice program on your computer, the synthesizer reads aloud the text on your computer monitor. It tells you what actions are taking place on screen: where the cursor is, what text is highlighted and other essential computer activities.

Apps and hardware

Smartphones and tablets now offer built-in accessibility features at little or no additional cost. Examples include text enlargement, contrast enhancement, zoom and voice command. These features

TABLETS AND ELECTRONIC READERS (E-READERS)

A common goal among people with low vision is to be able to read. For many people with low vision, enlarging text size is the best way to read more effectively. Traditionally, this meant relying on magnifiers or large-print books. Tablets and e-readers are changing that.

Tablets are minicomputers that can display electronic books, web pages, emails and other reading material. They come in various sizes and can be adapted so that all text is enlarged. You also can temporarily zoom in on text by "swiping" the display. Some tablets can display white text on a black background — rather than the traditional black text on a white background — which makes reading more comfortable for longer periods of time.

E-readers are about the same size as a tablet, but they tend to be lighter in weight than a tablet, and they hold their battery charge longer. They're primarily used for reading, as compared with tablets which can surf the web, return emails and download all kinds of apps. If you primarily read books, an e-reader may be a very inexpensive option.

Check with your low-vision technology specialist to decide which device may be right for you. Before you buy any device, ask questions and evaluate all of the available features. Make sure the device you're considering will meet your needs.

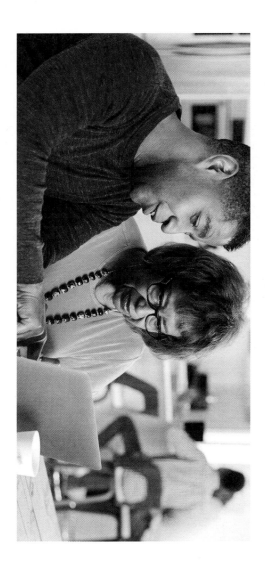

allow you to ask a number of devices to do things such as read your last text, state the time, send a message or make a grocery list.

In addition to built-in features, there are hundreds of apps that can be installed onto smartphones and tablets to help you perform tasks and recognize written words, colors, currency and more.

Head-worn technology

This is one of the fastest growing areas in low-vision technology. These devices, which you wear on your head, contain magnification capabilities to help with distance viewing. Cost can be a drawback, and it's not recommended that you walk with them on. Expect to hear more about this up-and-coming technology.

TAKING ACTION

People cope with the challenges of low vision in different ways. If you feel disappointed, frustrated, angry or sad about your vision loss, that's perfectly normal. Allow yourself some time to grieve.

Depression, however, is different from grieving, and having low vision increases the chance of experiencing depression. Signs and symptoms of depression can include loss of interest in activities, changes in sleep and eating patterns, irritability, and anxiety. If you are experiencing any of these, talk to your doctor.

If you're comfortable doing so, be open and honest with the people who love you most about your vision loss and how you feel. Let your family and friends know how they can help you, and when you don't need their help. Tell them if they're doing too much. People around you want to help, but they need your guidance.

Don't be afraid to reach out to individuals who can help you. Consider talking with a counselor or joining a support group for people with vision loss. This is a great way to engage with people with similar experiences, and to gain encouragement, advice and practical tips.

Focus on what you can do to make daily functioning easier. Taking action helps decrease anxiety and it provides you with added control and strength to cope with new circumstances.

Many people successfully overcome the challenges of low vision and continue to live independent and fulfilling lives.

Index

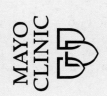